Field Guide to Clinical Dermatology

David H. Frankel, M.D.
North American Editor
The Lancet
New York, New York

Assistant Clinical Professor of Dermatology
Mount Sinai School of Medicine
New York, New York

 LIPPINCOTT WILLIAMS & WILKINS
A **Wolters Kluwer** Company
Philadelphia · Baltimore · New York · London
Buenos Aires · Hong Kong · Sydney · Tokyo

Acquisitions Editor: Richard Winters
Developmental Editor: Mary Beth Murphy
Production Editor: Jonathan Geffner
Manufacturing Manager: Tim Reynolds
Compositor: Maryland Composition

© 1999 by LIPPINCOTT WILLIAMS & WILKINS
530 Walnut Street
Philadelphia, PA 19106-3780 USA
www.LWW.com

Printed and bound in China

Library of Congress Cataloging-in-Publication Data

Field guide to clinical dermatology / [edited by] David H. Frankel.
    p.   cm.
  Includes index.
  ISBN 0-7817-1730-2
    1. Skin—Diseases Handbooks, manuals, etc, 2. Primary care
(Medicine) Handbooks, manuals, etc.   I. Frankel, David H.
  [DNLM: 1. Skin Diseases Handbooks.   WR 39 F453 1999]
RL74.F54   1999
616.5—dc21
DNLM/DLC
for Library of Congress   99-22603
                                                              CIP

Care has been taken to confirm the accuracy of the information presented and
to describe generally accepted practices. However, the authors, editor, and
publisher are not responsible for errors or omissions or for any consequences
from application of the information in this book and make no warranty, ex-
pressed or implied, with respect to the currency, completeness, or accuracy of
the contents of the publication. Application of this information in a particular
situation remains the professional responsibility of the practitioner.

The authors, editor, and publisher have exerted every effort to ensure that
drug selection and dosage set forth in this text are in accordance with current
recommendations and practice at the time of publication. However, in view of
ongoing research, changes in government regulations, and the constant flow of
information relating to drug therapy and drug reactions, the reader is urged to
check the package insert for each drug for any change in indications and
dosage and for added warnings and precautions. This is particularly important
when the recommended agent is a new or infrequently employed drug. Unless
specifically stated, most of the dosages in this book are for adult patients. Adjustments to these dosages must be made when treating children.

Some drugs and medical devices presented in this publication have Food
and Drug Administration (FDA) clearance for limited use in restricted research
settings. It is the responsibility of the health care provider to ascertain the FDA
status of each drug or device planned for use in their clinical practice.

10 9 8 7 6 5 4

Dedication

*This book is written in memory of
Charles Hohner and James Knox,
my English teachers.*

It is to honor my parents.

And it is dedicated to Annie.

Contents

Guide to the Book

IV. Bumps

A. Bumps you think may be cancer

B. Skin-colored bumps

VIII. Hair loss

IX. Procedures and supplies

Contributing Authors

Jeffrey P. Callen, M.D.   *Professor, Department of Medicine (Dermatology); Chief, Division of Dermatology, University of Louisville, 310 East Broadway, Louisville, Kentucky 40202*

John T. Crissey, M.D.   *Clinical Professor, Department of Medicine (Dermatology), University of Southern California, School of Medicine, 1975 Zonal Avenue, Los Angeles, California 90033; Attending Dermatologist, Department of Medicine (Dermatology), Los Angeles County–University of Southern California Medical Center, 1200 North State Street, Los Angeles, California 90033*

David H. Frankel, M.D.   *North American Editor, The Lancet, 655 Avenue of the Americas, New York, New York 10010; Assistant Clinical Professor of Dermatology, Mount Sinai School of Medicine, One Gustave L Levy Place, New York, New York 10029*

Charles A. Gropper, M.D.   *Assistant Clinical Professor of Dermatology, Department of Dermatology, Mount Sinai School of Medicine, 1 Gustave L. Levy Place, New York, New York 10029; Chief, Department of Dermatology, Bronx Veterans Affairs Medical Center, St. Barnabas Hospital, 130 West Kingsbridge Road, Bronx, New York 10468*

David J. Leffell, M.D.   *Professor, Departments of Dermatology and Surgery, Yale University School of Medicine; P.O. Box 208059; New Haven, Connecticut 06510; Attending Dermatologist, Chief, Section of Dermatologic Surgery and Cutaneous Oncology, Yale–New Haven Hospital, 20 York Street, New Haven, Connecticut 06510*

Larry E. Millikan, M.D.   *Professor and Chairman, Department of Dermatology, Tulane University Medical Center, 1430 Tulane Avenue, TB-36, New Orleans, Louisiana 70112; Chairman, Department of Dermatology, Tulane University Hospital and Clinic, 1415 Tulane Avenue, New Orleans, Louisiana 70112*

Lawrence Charles Parish, M.D. *Clinical Professor of Dermatology and Cutaneous Biology, Director, Jefferson Center for International Dermatology, Jefferson Medical College, Thomas Jefferson University, 1819 JFK Boulevard, Suite 465, Philadelphia, Pennsylvania 19103; and Chief, Department of Dermatology, Frankfort Hospital, Red Lion and Knights Roads, Philadelphia, Pennsylvania 19114*

Andrew J. Scheman, M.D. *Associate Professor of Clinical Dermatology, Department of Dermatology, Northwestern University Medical Center, 222 East Superior Avenue, 3rd floor, Chicago, Illinois 60611*

James C. Shaw, M.D. *Associate Professor of Clinical Medicine, Section of Dermatology, University of Chicago, 5841 South Maryland Avenue, Chicago, Illinois 60637; Chief, Section of Dermatology, University of Chicago Hospitals, 5841 South Maryland Avenue, Chicago, Illinois 60637*

Preface

This book is for primary-care practitioners. It is meant as a working manual, to be carried and used daily. It is deliberately long on direct, clinical content and short on pathogenesis and etiology. I hope it helps.

The medication dosages given in this book are for adult patients, unless otherwise noted. The dosages must therefore be adjusted for pediatric patients.

The Table of Contents and the Guide to the Book organize the text. I know it is a bit unorthodox. However, as an internist and dermatologist who has always practiced among primary-care professionals, I find that the standard dermatology algorithms are often a bit too long and confusing to be easily learned. I have therefore tried to organize the contents to reflect the predominance of two simple categories: what the patient says (e.g., "it itches"), or what you see (e.g., a red rash).

Of course, itch is subjective, red rashes scale, scaling rashes are red, and no algorithm is perfect. Therefore, only the predominant symptom or sign is the one that gets the title in the Guide to the Book. Please read the entire Guide to the Book. Most of the skin diseases you will see are listed there.

David H. Frankel, M.D.
Brooklyn, New York
October, 1998

Acknowledgments

I am grateful to the contributing authors of this book. All are practicing dermatologists who have spent much of their careers teaching dermatology to primary-care colleagues. Their enthusiasm and patience were constant, despite my unending demands for edits and re-edits. Thanks also to Richard Winters, my editor at Lippincott Williams & Wilkins, for his wise and careful guidance, and to Mary Beth Murphy, a developmental editor whose expertise took a thousand pieces and made a book. Thanks also to Jonathan Geffner, who polished the pages. I am fortunate to have enjoyed many years of kindness and support from *The Lancet*, and I am indebted to my friends and colleagues there.

CHAPTER 1

Proper Use of Topical Corticosteroids

Andrew J. Scheman, M.D.

WARNING

It is unusual to begin a pharmacology or formulary section with a warning. Warnings are generally reserved for the end. But because topical corticosteroids often cause serious local side effects when used improperly and because prescriptions are sometimes given in a cavalier manner, it is worth describing pitfalls at the outset.

Local side effects of steroid use can be permanent, disfiguring, and very distressing. Skin atrophied from topical corticosteroids appears thin, transparent, shiny, hypopigmented, and telangiectatic (Fig. 1-1). Striae may develop. These changes are especially noticeable and distressing on the face. Other high-risk areas prone to steroid atrophy are

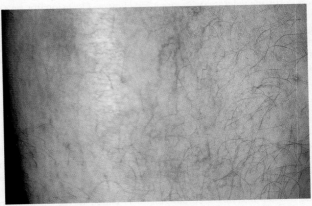

FIGURE 1. Atrophy from topical corticosteroids presents as thin, hypopigmented, telangiectatic skin.

intertriginous areas, such as the groin, axillae, neck, and intergluteal cleft.

It is worth remembering that topical corticosteroids may cause the same systemic side effects as oral corticosteroids. This is especially true in children, in whom the high ratio of skin surface area to body weight makes treatment of even relatively small areas of the skin more problematic.

Patients—or their family members—often use whatever cream is in the medicine cabinet. It is not unusual for a patient with acne to use a super-potent topical corticosteroid on the cheek or nose, believing that "one cream is just as good as another." Therefore, it is wise to prescribe only the amount that the patient needs immediately and to limit refills.

Although it sounds simplistic, patients on potent topical medications need follow-up no less than patients taking oral medications. Proper and timely adjustments of therapy to less (or more) potent preparations hastens relief from skin disease and limits the potential for untoward effects.

AVOIDING TOPICAL CORTICOSTEROID SIDE EFFECTS IN HIGH-RISK AREAS

Unfortunately, we all encounter instances in which a dermatitis on the face, groin, axillae, or intergluteal folds, or on a child does not respond to lowest potent agents. As will be discussed, low- or medium-potent topical corticosteroids that are nonfluorinated can be effective in this situation; desonide 0.05%, and, if a more potent agent is needed, hydrocortisone valerate 0.2%, are good choices. Occasionally, an even stronger preparation is needed. Mometasone furoate 0.1% is the only high potent topical corticosteroid ointment that is nonfluorinated. Caution is still in order, however. Although the use of nonfluorinated topical corticosteroids reduces the likelihood of side effects, it does not eliminate them.

TOPICAL CORTICOSTEROIDS ARE GROUPED BY STRENGTH

The list of topical corticosteroids has many chemical names that may be unfamiliar to you, and prednisone—probably the most commonly used systemic corticosteroid—is missing. This is because prednisone, like most systemic corticosteroids, is weak as an ointment or cream. When a fluorinated side chain is added to the basic steroid molecule, these glucocorticoids are effective as topical agents. Unfortunately, the fluorinated side chains also increase the potential for side effects. Indeed, many of today's topical corticosteroids can be dangerous, when they are used incorrectly.

The strength of a topical corticosteroid is measured by its ability to produce vasoconstriction, the Stoughton assay. The more vasoconstriction that occurs, the more potent is the steroid. On the basis of the vasoconstriction model, topical corticosteroids are divided into seven categories. Class 1 is the strongest, and class 7 is the weakest. For the purposes of this book, we label only five groups: (a) "super-potent," (b) "high-potent," (c) "medium-potent," (d) "low-potent," and (e) "lowest-potent/over the counter."

The strength of a topical corticosteroid is related to the potency of the steroid molecule. However, it is also related to the base, or vehicle, in which it is compounded. Ointments are often stronger than creams. Generic products may be a bit weaker than their branded "equivalents," but they are often considerably cheaper.

WHAT THE POTENCY GROUPS MEAN IN PRACTICE

Super-potent topical corticosteroids must be used with great caution. These fluorinated agents should be used only for limited eruptions (less than 10% of the body) on non–high-risk areas. They should not be used for more than 2 to 3 weeks or on children at all. After the acute eruption has been brought under control, it is wise to switch to a lower-strength preparation for maintenance therapy.

High-potent topical corticosteroids are usually fluorinated. Their use should be limited to small eruptions and not used on high-risk areas or on children. However, high-potent preparations can be used for longer periods of time than the super-potent products can and are indicated for maintenance therapy in severe, localized inflammatory skin problems. Again, their use must be closely supervised.

Medium-potent, **fluorinated** topical corticosteroids are used to control severe, widespread inflammatory dermatoses or to treat less severe, localized conditions. Medium-potent, **nonfluorinated** agents can be used for severe dermatoses of the face, groin, axilla, and intergluteal cleft, and on children.

Low-potent, **fluorinated** topical corticosteroids are used for moderately severe, inflammatory widespread dermatoses. Low-potent **nonfluorinated** agents are safer on the high-risk areas and on children.

Lowest-potent and over-the-counter preparations can be used on the high-risk areas and on children. Although hydrocortisone 2.5% would seem to be much stronger than hydrocortisone 1%, it is only marginally so. The 2.5% preparation is available by prescription only. Hydrocortisone 1% is the weakest topical corticosteroid that seems to be clinically effective; hydrocortisone 0.5% is of little benefit. Both are available over the counter.

A note of warning: some compounded products can surprise you. Lotrisone cream, one of the most widely prescribed topical medications for fungal infections, contains betamethasone dipropionate 0.05% in addition to the antifungal agent, clotrimazole. Another "antifungal," Mycolog II, contains triamcinolone acetonide 0.1% in addition to the antifungal nystatin. Even though these agents are often regarded as antifungals alone, they should not be used on high-risk areas or on children because they contain strong and potentially harmful fluorinated corticosteroids.

CHOOSING THE VEHICLE: OINTMENT, CREAM, OR SOLUTION?

An *ointment* is a heavy, occlusive, non–water-containing vehicle, which provides significant moisturization. **Creams** are emulsions of oil and water that are less moisturizing and dissolve more rapidly into the skin than ointment. Creams that are predominantly oil (oil-based) provide more moisturization than those that are predominantly water (water-based); oil-free creams are the least moisturizing. *Solutions* are liquid forms of topical corticosteroid in which the liquid vehicle is usually alcohol, water, or propylene glycol.

For dry skin conditions such as chronic atopic dermatitis, an ointment is best. For inflammatory dermatoses in which dry skin does not play a major role, such as contact dermatitis, creams are best. For oily dermatoses such as seborrheic dermatitis or for inflammatory conditions in areas of thick hair growth, solutions are best. Solutions can also be used on the face underneath cosmetics. Although some solutions are classified as super-, high- or medium-potent solutions, they are relatively safe to use long-term on the scalp. However, it is wise to examine the scalp periodically to make sure atrophy does not develop.

APPLICATION SCHEDULE AND AMOUNT TO DISPENSE

Topical corticosteroids are used twice daily. The amount dispensed varies by body habitus, but a rough measure for dispensing is shown in Table 1-1. See Appendix for a list of topical agents and their brand names.

TABLE 1–1. *Guidelines for Dispensing topical corticosteroids*

Location	Amount Dispensed (2× daily for 1 week)[a]
Face or neck	15 g
Chest or back	45 g
Hands (both)	15 g
Arm (one)	30 g
Feet (both)	30 g
Leg (one)	60 g
Entire body	180–240 g

[a] For children, reduce the amount dispensed proportional to adult body size.

APPENDIX 1. *Topical Corticosteroid Agents*

Strength	Brand
Ointments	
Super-potent	
Augmented betamethasone dipropionate 0.05%[a]	Diprolene
Clobetasol propionate 0.05%	Temovate
Diflorasone diacetate 0.05%[a]	Psorcon
Halobetasol propionate 0.05%[a]	Ultravate
High-potent	
Fluocinonide 0.05%	Lidex
Mometasone furoate 0.1%[a,b]	Elocon
Desoximetasone 0.25%	Topicort
Betamethasone dipropionate 0.05%	Diprosone
Medium-potent	
Betamethasone valerate 0.1%	Beta-val
Hydrocortisone valerate 0.2%[b]	Westcort
Triamcinolone acetonide 0.1%	Aristocort
Low-potent	
Desonide 0.05%[b]	DesOwen, Tridesilon
Triamcinolone acetonide 0.025%	Aristocort, Kenalog
Lowest-potent/over the counter	
Hydrocortisone 2.5%[b]	Hytone
Hydrocortisone 1.0%[b]	Over-the-counter
Creams	
Super-potent	
Clobetasol propionate 0.055%	Temovate
Halobetasol propionate 0.05%[a]	Ultravate
High-potent	
Augmented betamethasone dipropionate 0.05%[a]	Diprolene
Desoximetasone 0.25%	Topicort
Diflorasone diacetate 0.05%	Florone, Psorcon
Fluocinonide 0.05%	Lidex
Medium-potent	
Mometasone furoate 0.1%[a,b]	Elocon
Hydrocortisone valerate 0.2%[b]	Westcort
Triamcinolone acetonide 0.1%	Aristocort, Kenalog
Low-potent	
Desonide 0.05%[a]	DesOwen, Tridesilon
Fluocinolone acetonide 0.01%	Synalar
Lowest-potent/over the counter	
Hydrocortisone 2.5%[a]	Hytone
Hydrocortisone 1.0%[a]	Over-the-counter

APPENDIX 1. *(Continued)*

Solutions

Super-potent

Clobetasol propionate 0.05%	Temovate

High-potent

Fluocinonide 0.05%	Lidex

Medium-potent

Betamethasone valerate 0.01%	Betatrex
Betamethasone dipropionate 0.05%	Diprosone

Low-potent

Fluocinolone acetonide 0.025%	Synalar

Lowest-potent/over-the-counter

Hydrocortisone 1.0%[b]	Over-the-counter

Dozens of prescription topical corticosteroids are on the market, and new ones keep emerging. As a rule, generic preparations are far less expensive than branded products. Therefore, many of the products listed are generic preparations, although brand names are given for the sake of convenience.

[a] Not available in generic.
[b] Nonfluorinated.

CHAPTER 2

Atopic Dermatitis (ICD-9 691.8)

Lawrence Charles Parish, M.D.

SYMPTOMS AND SIGNS

The hallmark of atopic dermatitis (AD) is itching, which can be severe. AD is characterized by redness, scaling, and lichenification. In adults, it most commonly occurs in the antecubital and popliteal fossae (Figs. 2-1 and 2-2) and on the nape of the neck. Because there is no true primary lesion, patients with AD often present solely with itching or so-called "sensitive skin." As the skin is scratched or rubbed to obtain relief, it may show excoriations, vesiculation, and crusting. Secondary bacterial infection of the skin is common.

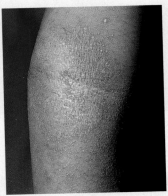

FIGURE 1. Atopic dermatitis. Antecubital erythema and lichenification is a hallmark of the disease.

Presentation of AD is variable, depending on the age of the patient. In infants and children, the redness and scaling may be on the extensor surfaces, face, or trunk. Infantile AD may be short-lived or may be a prodrome to lifelong dermatitis. As the child grows older, the traditional flexor areas become involved.

AD patients often have hyperlinear palms (Fig. 2-3) and infraorbital creases, so-called Dennie-Morgan folds. Rubbing of the lips creates cracking and surrounding erythema, known as the **furrowed mouth syndrome.** In older patients or during times of quiescence, the only manifestations of AD may be dryness and scaling—erythema crackle.

Associated conditions include pityriasis alba, in which there are irregular patches of scaling and hypopigmentation, and **keratosis pilaris**

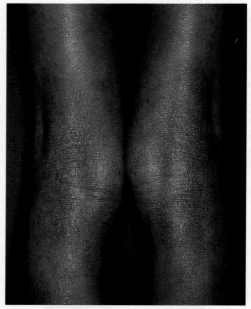

FIGURE 2. Atopic dermatitis. Typical appearance in the popliteal fossae with postinflammatory hyperpigmentation.

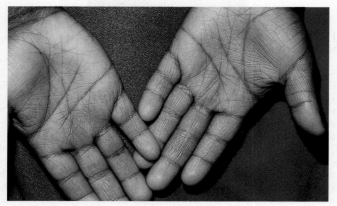

FIGURE 3. Hyperlinear palms are a clue to the diagnosis of atopic dermatitis.

(KP), the almost physiologic hyperkeratotic accentuation of hair follicles on the lateral and posterior upper arms and on the anterior thighs (Fig. 2-4). Keratosis pilaris presents as firm red or skin-colored papules, giving a "sandpaper" feel to the area. African-American patients may also have perifollicular accentuation like goose flesh.

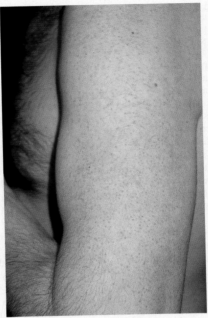

FIGURE 4. Keratosis pilaris. Hyperkeratotic follicular papules on extensor aspect of the upper arms or on the anterior thighs feel like sandpaper and respond to lactic acid cream or lotion.

DIFFERENTIAL DIAGNOSIS

Seborrheic dermatitis is usually limited to the scalp, glabella, and perinasal area. Contact dermatitis, especially when it is on the hands, can mimic AD. The history helps in achieving a diagnosis. Neurodermatitis has a similar morphology and sometimes more varied distribution, but the distinguishing feature is the lack of atopic history—asthma, allergic rhinitis, or eczema in the patient or in a relative. Redness and scaling on the feet may suggest tinea pedis; however, children rarely have a dermatophyte infection, and the lack of interdigital involvement rules out a fungal infection.

How to Make the Diagnosis

Although AD may result in eosinophilia or elevated immunoglobulin E (IgE) levels, the diagnosis is made by observation and the personal or family history of atopy. Hyperlinear palms and Dennie-Morgan fold are helpful clues. White dermatographism, in which stroking the skin gives a raised white line, is common.

TREATMENT

The most important aspect of therapy is to "put the skin to rest" by avoiding irritants. Soap should be limited to the critical areas—hands, face, axillae, and groin. Excessively hot water is also destructive to the skin. Patients will want to bathe daily, but extensive soaking may aggravate their skin. Short, lukewarm showers are acceptable.

Topical corticosteroids are needed for long periods of time. Therefore, high-potent and super-potent ointments or creams should be limited to flares, and medium-potent or low-potent agents should be used for maintenance. Oral corticosteroids should be reserved for severe flares. Prednisone, 30 mg daily for 10 days, may break the cycle. Colloidal baths initially reduce itching, whereas oral antihistamines relieve pruritus but do not affect the natural course of this chronic dermatitis.

Patients should be encouraged to use unscented moisturizers. Creams or ointments are more effective than lotions and should be applied immediately after showering to limit irritation and drying, which inevitably results from soap and water. This is especially important in winter. Remember that the sensitivity to wool of patients with AD carries over into lanolin-based products. Lipid-free products are safest. In hot, humid weather, secondary bacterial infection may require a course of antistaphylococcal oral antimicrobial agents such as erythromycin, 250 mg three times daily for 7 to 10 days.

Keratosis pilaris responds to lactic acid 12% cream or lotion applied twice daily.

PROGNOSIS

There is no way to know how long AD will last. Often, infants and children have AD that never returns in later years. Other patients develop AD in middle age; still others have severe AD for most of their lives. Sometimes AD surfaces only for periods during adulthood. If patients attend carefully to proper skin care, they are less likely to have severe disease if—or when—the condition recurs.

CHAPTER 3

Contact Dermatitis (ICD-9 692.9)

Lawrence Charles Parish, M.D.

SYMPTOMS AND SIGNS

Contact dermatitis itches and burns. It is characterized by redness, which can progress to vesiculation, oozing, weeping, scaling, and fissuring. After several days of itching and rubbing, the areas may develop secondary bacterial infection with purulence and crusting. Sometimes the reaction is so intense that swelling occurs at the contact site and dermatitis occurs at distant sites. The latter phenomenon is called an **id reaction.** Contact dermatitis may be divided into two groups: irritant and allergic.

Irritant contact dermatitis occurs every time the patient comes into contact with the substance. This irritant can develop in a few minutes or in several hours. Any person is subject to irritant dermatitis if he or she is in contact with an irritating substance long enough. The duration of exposure required to produce dermatitis varies. Perhaps the most common contact irritant is soap, especially in the wintertime when skin is already dry and irritated. Other common irritants include detergents, cutting oils, solvents, and cement.

Allergic contact dermatitis develops within 24 to 48 hours after exposure to an allergen to which the patient has previously been sensitized. Rhus dermatitis, caused by poison oak, poison ivy, or poison sumac, is the prototypical allergic response. The dermatitis lasts for 10 to 20 days because the rhus oil becomes embedded in the skin. A clue to the diagnosis is its linear pattern. Other common contact allergens include nickel, neomycin, rubber (latex), paraphenylenediamine, lanolin, topical anesthetics, topical antihistamines, and fragrances. It is worth remembering that most metal jewelry contains nickel, even when it is advertised as "solid gold" (Fig. 3-1). Topical neomycin is the most common cause of iatrogenic allergic contact dermatitis.

DIFFERENTIAL DIAGNOSIS

Contact dermatitis is often distinctive because of its localization. Occasionally, it may be confused with atopic dermatitis limited to the antecubital or popliteal fossae or with nummular dermatitis scattered on the body. Because dermatitis on the hands may be nondescript, the term **hand dermatitis** is used to cover a number of dermatitides: atopic, contact, and psoriatic.

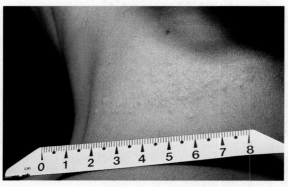

FIGURE 1. Nickel-causing allergic contact dermatitis from solid gold necklace.

HOW TO MAKE THE DIAGNOSIS

The history is most important. If the patient recognizes this every time he or she has contact with a particular item, then the etiologic battle is won. Sometimes, the offending agent is more difficult to locate, and patch testing is necessary. This involves placing a series of chemicals on the skin, usually the back, covering the applications with a type of nonirritating and nonallergenic dressing such as paper tape and keeping the area covered for 2 to 3 days. Reaction at the site of the chemical helps confirm the diagnosis.

TREATMENT

Eliminating the contactant is crucial, whereas topical corticosteroid ointments and creams are most helpful in reducing the dermatitis. The strength of the steroid depends on the severity of the dermatitis. With a severe reaction, such as a reaction to paraphenylenediamine in hair dye or to poison ivy, oral prednisone, 40 to 60 mg per day for 10 days, may be needed in addition to high-potent or super-potent topical corticosteroids.

PROGNOSIS

The dermatitis usually clears within a few days after the elimination of the contactant. Reexposure, particularly chronic reexposure, leads to chronic dermatitis and lichenification.

CHAPTER 4

Scabies (ICD-9 133.0)

Lawrence Charles Parish, M.D.

SYMPTOMS AND SIGNS

Scabies causes severe itching, especially at night, when there are fewer distractions. (It is sometimes called the "7-year itch" because it probably lasts 7 years without treatment.) The eruption is characterized by small, 2- to 5-mm red papules that are predominantly found in intertriginous or warm and protected areas such as the finger webs (Fig. 4-1), inframammary areas, and axillae. It is caused by the mite, *Sarcoptes scabei.* The pathognomonic lesion is the burrow, a brownish, irregular line with scaling at one end and sometimes a vesicle at the other end. Unfortunately, the burrow is often hard to find. Another common site is the penis. Lesions can also appear on the trunk and extremities, but rarely on the face except in children or in immune-compromised patients. The papules sometimes are eczematized and secondarily infected as the result of scratching to alleviate the marked nocturnal itching.

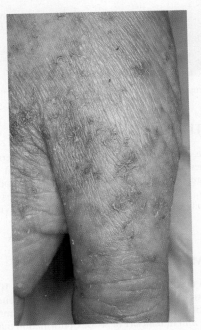

FIGURE 1. Scabies causing burrows in web spaces of the hand.

The presentation of scabies can vary. Infants and elderly can have red papules scattered over the entire body. Crusted scabies represents a severe infestation that occurs in immune-compromised patients (Fig. 4-2). "Scabies incognito" occurs when the patient has been applying topical corticosteroids, which impede the inflammatory process but still allow the mites to proliferate.

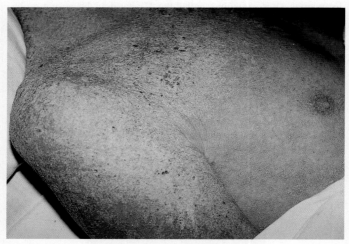

FIGURE 2. Crusted scabies in a patient with AIDS.

DIFFERENTIAL DIAGNOSIS

Scabies can be confused with folliculitis and neurodermatitis. Insect bites from other arthropods can look like scabies, but penile lesions confirm the presence of scabies. Canine scabies produces clusters of red papules, usually on the abdomen, but no mites are found on the human skin. Crusted scabies can be confused with eczema or psoriasis.

HOW TO MAKE THE DIAGNOSIS

A recent lesion is scraped, the material is treated with 10% potassium hydroxide solution to dissolve the keratin, and the specimen is studied under light microscopy. The mite measures 0.4 × 0.3 mm for females and 0.2 × 0.15 mm in males (Fig. 4-3). Confirmation may be difficult to obtain if the patient has washed conscientiously with soap.

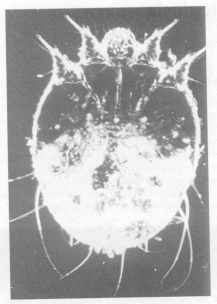

FIGURE 3. *Sarcoptes scabei* seen under the microscope.

TREATMENT

Permethrin cream 5% is applied from head to toes for 12 hours before being washed off. A second choice is lindane lotion 1%, applied from the neck to the toes for a 12-hour period before being washed off. Lindane should not be used in infants or in pregnant women. Ivermectin, 200 µg/kg given once, is used as an oral treatment in some countries. To prevent undertreatment or recurrence, topical treatments must be applied to all areas including in the umbilicus and under the fingernails. Symptomatic relief is given with high-potent to super-potent topical corticosteroid ointment or cream. Pruritus can persist even weeks beyond successful therapy.

Treatment should include close contacts and family members.

PROGNOSIS

When the application of cream or lotion is inadequate, the condition persists.

CHAPTER 5

Pediculosis (ICD-9 132.0 capitis; 132.2 pubis; 132.1 corporis)

Lawrence Charles Parish, M.D.

SYMPTOMS AND SIGNS

Pediculosis can be very pruritic. There are three forms in humans: pediculosis pubis caused by *Pthirus pubis*, pediculosis capitis caused by *Pediculus capitis*, and pediculosis corporis caused by *Pediculus corporis*.

Pediculosis capitis is found only in preadolescent children and almost never in African-American children, for unknown reasons. Scratching can cause a secondary bacterial infection. Crusting appears on the scalp, and excoriations appear on the neck and ears. Occipital and cervical lymph nodes are palpable. Live nits are whitish and shiny and found within 1 cm of the scalp (Fig. 5-1). Dead nits are dull and gray.

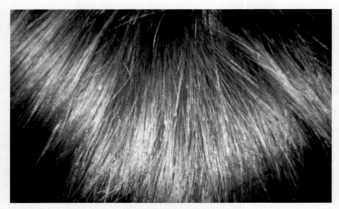

FIGURE 1. Pediculosis capitis with white, shiny nits.

Pediculosis pubis is caused by a crab-like organism; hence, "crab lice" infestation. The louse grasps the hair and bites the skin, often producing bluish macules 0.5 to 2.5 cm in diameter (maculae ceruleae). The nit is 3 to 4 mm in length. Although generally found on the pubic hairs, the crab louse attaches to hair on other parts of the body, such as the scalp or axilla. **Pediculosis ciliaris,** seen mostly in children, is due to pubic louse infestation of the eyelids.

Pediculosis corporis is caused by a larger louse that feeds on the skin but does not remain attached, preferring to reside in the seams of clothing. Intense itching leads to eczematization—**vagabonds' disease.** Body lice can transmit epidemic typhus (*Rickettsia prowazekii*), trench fever (*Bartonella quintana*), and louse-borne relapsing fever (*Borrelia recurrentis*).

DIFFERENTIAL DIAGNOSIS

Seborrheic dermatitis—"walking dandruff"—is scaling, and the scales do not stick to hair. It can be distinguished by its successful treatment with tar shampoo. Contact dermatitis and drug eruptions cause diffuse pruritus.

HOW TO MAKE THE DIAGNOSIS

Finding the live louse or nit on a hair shaft makes the diagnosis of head louse and pubic louse infestation. A hand lens is helpful in identifying the nit, which is attached to the hair shaft by a cementum (Fig. 5-2). Wood's light examination shows whitish fluorescence of the hair and the nits. Inspection of the patient's clothing, particularly the seams, will reveal body lice. Often, these diagnostic tips are absent, and a presumptive diagnosis is made on the basis of excoriations in typical areas.

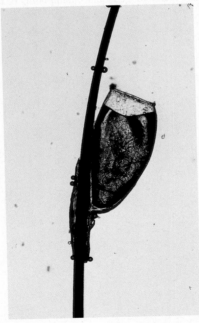

FIGURE 2. Nit attached to hair shaft seen with a hand lens.

TREATMENT

Both head lice and crab lice infestations can be treated with 5% permethrin or 1% lindane shampoo, applied for 10 minutes and repeated in a day or a week. (Lindane should not be used on infants or on pregnant women.) The nits can remain. Combing them out can be assisted by using white vinegar acid rinse.

Body lice infestation is managed by washing the clothes in hot water or disposing of them. The skin is then treated symptomatically with topical corticosteroid ointments or creams. The strength depends on the degree of itch; usually, medium-potent to high-potent creams are needed. Insecticides are not needed. Although live nits can live off of the skin for 1 or 2 days, they are sensitive enough to the temperature changes of daily living so that additional treatment is not necessary. Nits can transmit infestation in close contact so that treatment of household members and schoolmates is recommended.

PROGNOSIS

Treatment failure is due to inadequate shampooing or reinfestation.

CHAPTER 6

Dyshidrotic Eczema (ICD-9 705.81)

Lawrence Charles Parish, M.D.

SYMPTOMS AND SIGNS

Patients complain of itching or burning, which is sometimes intense. The hallmark of dyshidrotic eczema is deep-seated, clear blisters on the sides of the fingers (Fig. 6-1) and on the palms and soles. Because the epidermis is thicker in these areas, the blisters are deep and are often said to look like tapioca pudding. When they break, they leave collarettes of scale that last 2 to 3 weeks. Sometimes, there is oozing and crusting. Dyshidrotic eczema is sometimes associated with hyperhidrosis, atopic dermatitis, or contact dermatitis. Symptoms are worse in warm weather, but the condition may flare in the winter if the skin is dry. The disease is also called **pompholyx.**

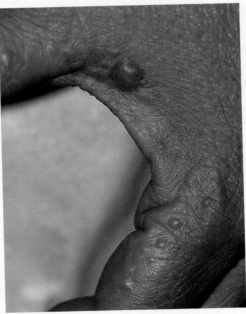

FIGURE 1. Pruritic vesicles on the sides of the fingers.

DIFFERENTIAL DIAGNOSIS

Atopic dermatitis and contact dermatitis are usually not limited to the sides of the fingers, although they can be present on only the palms or soles. Rarely, id reactions to dermatophytes or to bacteria mimic dyshidrosis. However, tinea pedis and tinea manuum are more disseminated on feet or hands and often more erythematous.

HOW TO MAKE THE DIAGNOSIS

The clinical presentation of dyshidrotic eczema suggests the diagnosis. Look especially for tapioca pudding–like vesicles.

TREATMENT

Medium-potent to super-potent topical corticosteroid creams or ointments bring acute conditions under control. Secondary bacterial infection may require oral erythromycin or cephalexin, 250 mg three to four times daily for 7 to 10 days. For weeping lesions, use compresses of Burows Solution in water 1:40 for 5 minutes three times daily. Addition of ice water to dilute the powder offers more relief. After the acute outbreak is relieved, a low-potent topical corticosteroid may be used to suppress the condition.

PROGNOSIS

Dyshidrosis waxes and wanes. Usually, acute attacks clear within 1 or 2 weeks of treatment, but occasionally it smolders for months.

CHAPTER 7

Stasis Dermatitis (ICD-9 454.1)

Lawrence Charles Parish, M.D.

SYMPTOMS AND SIGNS

Stasis dermatitis may initially cause an aching or gnawing feeling in the legs. Itching and burning may be intense enough to result in excoriations, secondary bacterial infection, and even an id reaction. An **id reaction** is a dermatitis that appears at a distant site on the body, usually the hands and arms. Stasis dermatitis occurs in older patients when venous or lymphatic return in the legs has been compromised. With increased extravasation of blood into the tissues, darkening becomes more permanent and soon erythema, scaling, and oozing appear (Fig. 7-1). Occasionally, the process leads to irregularly shaped ulcerations, known as **stasis ulcers** (see Chapter 70).

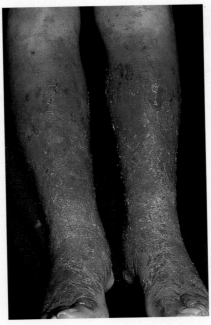

FIGURE 1. Stasis dermatitis causes erythema, scaling, and sometimes oozing on the lower legs.

DIFFERENTIAL DIAGNOSIS

Stasis dermatitis is limited to legs, but the eruption can mimic contact dermatitis and neurodermatitis. The former was common in the past with the use of topical anesthetics and ammoniated mercury; the latter was distinguished by patches of dermatitis being found elsewhere on the body.

HOW TO MAKE THE DIAGNOSIS

Patchy redness and scaling on the legs constitute the hallmark of stasis dermatitis until proved otherwise.

TREATMENT

High-potent or super-potent topical corticosteroid cream or ointment, applied twice daily for several weeks or months, is needed to resolve the acute inflammation. Secondary infection can be treated with erythromycin, 250 mg three times daily by mouth for 7 to 10 days. Patients should also elevate the legs and wear support hosiery.

PROGNOSIS

Stasis dermatitis is a chronic condition that smolders for years. With appropriate therapy, it can be controlled.

CHAPTER 8

Pruritis and Excoriations With No Primary Skin Lesions

(generalized pruritus ICD-9 698.9;

lichen simplex chronicus ICD-9 698.3; prurigo nodularis ICD-9

698.3)

Jeffrey P. Callen M.D.

SYMPTOMS AND SIGNS

Many patients complain of pruritus but have either no discernible rash or a rash that is initiated by scratching.

One of the more common causes of pruritus is dry skin, particularly in the elderly and during the winter. It is worsened with bathing and harsh soaps. Patients may have no visible skin changes, or they may develop excoriated, eczematous patches, which can become impetiginized.

When no visible changes are present, an attempt should be made to elicit **dermatographism,** the appearance of a hive from stroking of the skin (see Fig. 15-2). Dermatographism is more common in patients with urticaria.

Patients without obvious skin diseases should also be evaluated for systemic disease. Common causes are renal disease (uremia and hemodialysis-related), hepatobiliary disease (primary biliary cirrhosis and cholestatic problems), thyroid disease (both hypothyroidism and hyperthyroidism), diabetes mellitus, hematologic disease (polycythemia vera), malignancy (lymphoma), and infection with the HIV virus.

Drugs associated with pruritus include antibiotics, opiates, bleomycin, angiotensin-converting enzyme inhibitors, diuretics, sulfonylureas, estrogens, antithyroid agents, and anticoagulants.

Two conditions initiated by constant scratching are **prurigo nodularis** and **lichen simplex chronicus**. Large, firm, hyperpigmented nodules of prurigo nodularis often develop in crops on the arms and legs (Fig. 8-1). Lichen simplex chronicus is a single and favorite area of intense itching and habitual scratching. Lichenification is the hallmark sign, but the lesions are also notably red and scaling. Common sites are the lower legs, neck, wrists, and ankles (Fig. 8-2).

DIFFERENTIAL DIAGNOSIS

In patients with excoriations, causes such as scabies, eczemas, or dermatitis herpetiformis should be excluded. Patients with scabies have intense nocturnal pruritus; excoriations with burrows on the wrists, genitalia, and web spaces of the hands; and family members with symptoms. Dermatitis herpetiformis manifests as symmetric grouped excoriations, and occasionally vesicles, on the extensor surfaces such

23

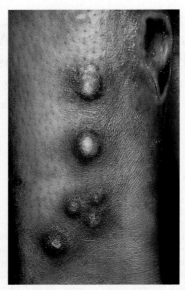

FIGURE 1. Prurigo nodularis, with multiple pruritic, hyperpigmented nodules on the arms also demonstrates a self-induced ulcer.

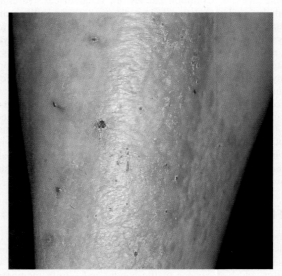

FIGURE 2. Lichen simplex chronicus develops in a single favorite area of scratching (the shin, in this patient).

as the the elbows or buttocks. Eczemas have typical distribution patterns and eventual lichenification.

HOW TO MAKE THE DIAGNOSIS

Scabies can be confirmed by skin scrapings. Patients with findings suggestive of dermatitis herpetiformis should have a punch biopsy of lesional skin for routine processing and perilesional normal-appearing skin for immunofluorescence microscopy. Systemic disease in patients is often evident by history. However, at a minimum, patients should have a physical examination and a complete blood count, liver, renal, and thyroid function tests, and a chest x-ray.

TREATMENT

General care of the patient with generalized pruritus involves application of emollients. Occasionally, a medium-potent corticosteroid cream or ointment is helpful for temporary relief. But if the itch is generalized, topical corticosteroids are impractical and can result in corticosteroid-related systemic toxicity from percutaneous absorption. Lotions containing 0.25% to 0.5% menthol or phenol, or 0.25% menthol in a medium-potency corticosteroid cream may give temporary relief. Oral antihistamines such as hydroxyzine, 10 to 25 mg, cyproheptadine 4 mg, or doxepin, 25 to 50 mg, should be taken before sleep and three to four times daily as needed. Nonsedating and mildly sedating antihistamines offer little benefit. Topical antihistamines are not recommended as they often cause contact dermatitis.

Pruritus due to an underlying systemic disease may cease once the underlying disease is successfully treated. For patients with renal disease, hepatobiliary disease, and HIV-associated pruritus, medically supervised ultraviolet B phototherapy may be helpful. Malignancy-associated pruritus abates with remission and reappears with relapse.

Prurigo nodularis and lichen simplex chronicus require high-potent to super-potent topical corticosteroid cream or ointment and encouraging, supportive care. These lesions can be stubborn.

PROGNOSIS

Prognosis depends on the cause. In idiopathic disease, there are no life-threatening consequences of generalized pruritus.

CHAPTER 9

Acne Vulgaris (ICD-9 706.1)

James C. Shaw, M.D.

SYMPTOMS AND SIGNS

Acne vulgaris is usually asymptomatic, although large nodular lesions can be tender. Affected patients usually present during adolescence with comedones, papules, pustules, nodules, or a combination. Closed comedones (whiteheads) and open comedones (blackheads) represent plugged hair follicles or "pores" and are small—1 to 3 mm in diameter. Their dark color is due to oxidation of surface keratin. Papules and pustules are 2 to 4 mm in diameter and have a slightly erythematous base (Fig. 9-1).

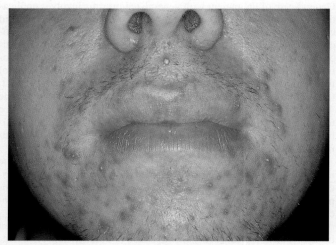

FIGURE 1. Acne vulgaris. Inflammatory papules and pustules.

Nodules are deeper erythematous lesions ranging from 6 to 20 mm in diameter (Fig. 9-2). Nodules occur on the face, neck, back, and chest. The term "cystic acne" has been abandoned because the lesions are not true cysts. "Severe nodular acne" is the preferred nomenclature. Acne is not limited to adolescence and can persist into adult years. It may even manifest for the first time in adulthood. This is especially common in women.

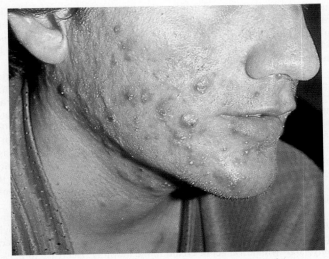

FIGURE 2. Nodular acne is the main indication for isotretinoin therapy.

DIFFERENTIAL DIAGNOSIS

Comedones due to chemical exposures (aromatic chlorinated hydrocarbons such as dioxin and herbicides) cause extensive face and neck lesions. Papules and pustules can be seen in rosacea, bacterial folliculitis or "steroid acne," which is caused by systemic or topical corticosteroids. Culture of a papule may be required to exclude bacterial folliculitis.

HOW TO MAKE THE DIAGNOSIS

Acne vulgaris is a clinical diagnosis. The presence of open comedones or closed comedones in an adolescent patient usually confirms it. If a patient presents with only pustules on the face, a bacterial culture may be required to exclude bacterial folliculitis.

TREATMENT

Patients must be told at the beginning of therapy that response to any treatment may take up to 6 weeks and that patience on their part (and on their doctor's part) will usually be rewarded. In general, it is helpful to advise acne patients that gentle washing once or twice daily is sufficient. Scrubs, abrasives, and alcohol-based toners/clarifiers often are irritating, especially when combined with topical acne medications, which can dry and inflame the skin. Washing does not cure acne. It merely washes off oils, dirt, makeup, and so on.

For patients with only comedonal disease, topical keratolytic agents are appropriate; tretinoin, azaleic acid 2% cream, adapalene 0.1% gel applied nightly on dry skin. Tretinoin comes in several strengths. Patients with sensitive skin should start with the least irritating, 0.025% cream. The strength can be increased to 0.05% to 0.1% cream if there is no response within 2 months, as long as the patient tolerates irritation that commonly complicates therapy. Gel formulation is more irritating but more effective (0.01% to 0.025%). Keratolytic agents are generally applied once daily, but can be used twice daily if tolerated. Sunscreens may prevent sun sensitivity caused by any of these agents.

Patients with superficial inflammatory papules require topical antimicrobial agents. These may be combined with keratolytics. Benzoyl peroxide–containing gels, creams, or washes should be applied once daily. Start with a 5% gel or cream in the morning. Decrease to 2.5% if this is too irritating, or increase to 10% as needed. Washes are best for large areas such as the back and chest. Clindamycin 1% or erythromycin 2% are supplied as lotion, solution, pledgets, or gel. Use lotions for dry skin and alcohol-based solution, pledgets or gel for oily skin. These should not be applied at the same time as benzoyl peroxide.

For moderately severe inflammatory acne, systemic antibiotics must be used for at least 1 to 3 months. Choices and doses include tetracycline 500 mg twice daily, doxycycline 50 to 100 mg twice daily, minocycline 100 mg daily, or erythromycin 250 mg four times daily or erythromycin ethylsuccinate 400 mg two to three times daily.

In patients with severe nodular acne, in recalcitrant cases, or when there is scarring, isotretinoin is the drug of choice. Standard dosing is 1 to 2 mg/kg daily for 4 to 6 months. Experience with isotretinoin and its complications is essential for safe use. The drug is contraindicated in women of childbearing age without adequate birth control measures and counseling. Two forms of contraception are recommended for women who do not choose abstinence.

Pretreatment blood work-up includes pregnancy testing, complete blood count, liver function studies, and lipid profile. These tests should be repeated monthly. Common side effects are cheilitis (90%) and elevated serum triglyceride levels (25%). Less common are conjunctivitis, xerosis, musculoskeletal pains, arthralgias, and hair thinning. Cheilitis is best treated with an ointment such as petroleum jelly. It is often helpful to advise patients to put petroleum jelly inside the nose at bedtime to prevent bleeding from a dry nasal mucosa. Sunscreens should be used daily because of photosensitivity.

PROGNOSIS

Most patients with adolescent acne improve spontaneously. Nonetheless, there may be severe and lifelong psychological effects. Patients with adult acne can continue to have episodic or persistent involvement for many years.

CHAPTER 10
Perioral Dermatitis (ICD 695.3)
Jeffrey P. Callen, M.D.

SIGNS AND SYMPTOMS

Although lesions of perioral dermatitis may burn or feel tender, most patients complain about their appearance rather than about specific symptoms. The disease is more common in women and usually occurs in early adulthood (25 to 35 years of age). Erythematous papules and pustules with minimal scale are the characteristic lesions (Fig. 10-1). This process is worsened by fluorinated topical corticosteroids or by fluorinated tartar control toothpastes.

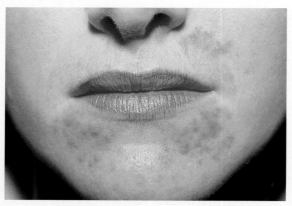

FIGURE 1. Perioral dermatitis. Erythematous perioral papules seen almost exclusively in young women.

DIFFERENTIAL DIAGNOSIS

Rosacea has more extensive facial lesions and greater amounts of flushing. Acne vulgaris has other types of lesions such as comedos and larger cysts, and patients are often younger. Contact dermatitis is pruritic and can often be linked to a specific agent. Seborrhea is scaly, is located on the central face, and has accompanying dandruff.

HOW TO MAKE THE DIAGNOSIS

The diagnosis is made by clinical examination. Punch biopsy or laboratory testing is rarely necessary. Patch testing excludes a contact dermatitis.

TREATMENT

A low-potent topical corticosteroid cream or ointment compounded with 1% precipitated sulfur is helpful. Alternatives include metronidazole 0.075% cream or gel, and topical clindamycin 2% or erythromycin 2% in lotions or gels. Oral tetracycline, 500 to 1,000 mg daily, is also helpful. The onset of effect, however, is delayed 4 to 6 weeks. Recalcitrant individual lesions may be injected with small amounts (less than 0.05 mL) of triamcinolone acetonide solution in a concentration of 3 mg/mL.

PROGNOSIS

Perioral dermatitis heals spontaneously, but this may take years to occur.

CHAPTER 11

Rosacea (ICD-9 695.3)

Larry E. Millikan, M.D.

SYMPTOMS AND SIGNS

The classic symptom of rosacea is flushing, although often this is lacking. Patients usually complain of a red nose or face. The condition is made worse by hot (temperature) or spicy foods or beverages, alcohol, and sunlight. The findings can be subtle and limited to merely mild telangiectasia and centrofacial erythema. More pronounced rosacea appears as acneiform facial papules, pustules, and frank ruddiness (Fig. 11-1). Some clinicians talk of the "rosacea oval," a vertical pattern of erythema from glabella to chin. Thickening and enlargement of nasal skin can cause the characteristic bulbous nose of rhinophyma, but this is rare. Northern European and Celtic patients are affected most. Eye diseases, such as conjunctivitis, blepharitis, episcleritis, or keratitis, are common complications of rosacea.

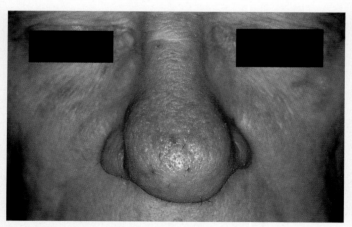

FIGURE 1. Rosacea. Note red nose with acneiform papules; telangiectasia is present on nose and cheeks.

DIFFERENTIAL DIAGNOSIS

Erythema from seborrheic dermatitis is accompanied by scaling on the scalp, nasal creases, and nasolabial folds. Acne vulgaris is not as often centrofacial or telangiectatic. Contact dermatitis will have a suggestive history and itching. Skin changes of systemic lupus erythematosus are malar and induced by sunlight.

HOW TO MAKE DIAGNOSIS

History—especially relationship to certain foods—genetic tendency, and centrofacial involvement are usually sufficient to make the diagnosis of rosacea.

TREATMENT

The traditional oral treatment is tetracycline, 500 mg twice daily; doxycycline, 100 mg twice daily, is an alternative. Metronidazole 0.075% gel or cream two to three times daily is often effective but may take several months to work. Rhinophyma can be treated by laser or electrosurgery. Eye symptoms should be evaluated by an ophthalmologist.

PROGNOSIS

Treatment usually provides symptomatic relief. It is not clear if early aggressive therapy impedes the rare progression to rhinophyma.

CHAPTER 12

Seborrheic Dermatitis (ICD-9 609.1)

Larry E. Millikan, M.D.

SYMPTOMS AND SIGNS

Seborrheic dermatitis (SD) of the face is often pruritic, but only mildly so. Itching in the scalp, however, is a common symptom. There is erythema and fine, branlike scaling on the forehead, nasolabial folds, around the ears and on the eyebrows or eyelids (Fig. 12-1). The scalp is often involved—common dandruff—as are presternal and intertriginous areas, such as the vault of the axilla and the groin. Seborrheic blepharitis is SD of the eyelids and margins. The condition can be florid in AIDS patients.

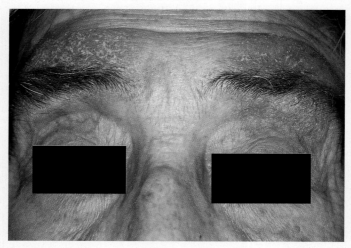

FIGURE 1. Seborrheic dermatitis. Erythema and fine, branlike scaling on eyebrows.

DIFFERENTIAL DIAGNOSIS

Psoriasis has a typical pattern of distribution on the elbows, knees, scalp, and nails. In tinea, lesions are more circumscribed and hyphae are seen under the microscope. The hallmark of candidiasis is intertriginous involvement. Contact dermatitis can be distinguished by history of offending agent and more pruritus. Rosacea patients have a history of flushing, and the centrofacial erythema is not accompanied by scales.

HOW TO MAKE DIAGNOSIS

Diagnosis of SD is made on clinical distribution and response to therapy. It is worthwhile to look for evidence of SD in all possible body sites.

TREATMENT

SD is a chronic and recurring condition, and patients may treat themselves without supervision for long periods. Therefore, use only low-potent topical corticosteroid ointments or creams. Antifungal creams of the imidazole or allylamine classes can also be effective but work more slowly. High-potent or super-potent corticosteroid solutions are safe on the scalp for long periods. Medicated shampoos should contain tar, zinc, sulfur, or salicylic acid. The antifungal shampoo, ketoconazole 2%, can be used twice weekly.

PROGNOSIS

SD often recurs in times of stress, either physical or emotional. Seborrheic blepharitis can lead to recurring infections of the eyelids, with hordeolum and conjunctivitis.

CHAPTER 13
Lupus Erythematosus (ICD-9 695.4)
Jeffrey P. Callen, M.D.

SIGNS AND SYMPTOMS

Cutaneous lupus erythematosus (LE) can be divided into chronic, sub-acute, and systemic forms. Patients may complain of photosensitivity, pruritic lesions, arthralgias, and myalgias.

Chronic cutaneous LE is most commonly manifested as **discoid LE** (DLE). Lesions of DLE are red with adherent scale, telangiectasia, follicular plugging, and dyspigmentation. Atrophy and scarring are characteristic (Fig. 13-1). Lesions occur most often on the head, neck, ears, scalp, arms, and upper chest and back. Less than 5% of patients with DLE have systemic manifestations of lupus.

Systemic LE (SLE) often presents as the classic, malar "butterfly" rash (Fig. 13-2). The rash is exacerbated by sun exposure or exposure to ultraviolet B (UVB) or ultraviolet A (UVA) from artificial light sources. Almost all patients with a butterfly rash have active SLE. **Subacute cutaneous LE** (SCLE) lesions are of at least two types: annular or papulosquamous. Both forms begin as red papules or plaques on sun-exposed skin, which eventually expand and form either rings or

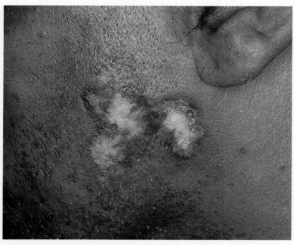

FIGURE 1. Discoid lupus erythematosus presents with sharply marginated atrophic plaques with central hypopigmentation and peripheral hyperpigmentation.

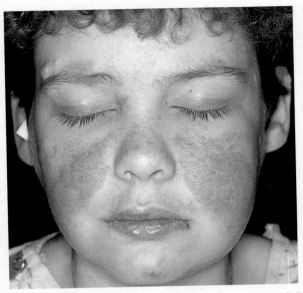

FIGURE 2. Systemic lupus erythematosus with classic malar "butterfly" erythema.

psoriasiform lesions. Annular lesions have central clearing. Papulosquamous lesions are scaling. About 50% of SCLE patients have evidence of systemic manifestations of lupus. SCLE is associated with Sjögren's syndrome, idiopathic thrombocytopenic purpura, cutaneous vasculitis, or deficiency of the second component of complement (C2d). It may be induced by a variety of drugs, most commonly hydrochlorothiazide and calcium channel blockers.

DIFFERENTIAL DIAGNOSIS

DLE and papulosquamous SCLE may simulate many other papulosquamous disorders. Psoriasis often has the classic knee, elbow, and scalp distribution. Lichen planus papules are violaceous, and oral lesions are common. Secondary syphilis involves the palms and soles. Dermatophytes do not preferentially infect sun-exposed skin, and papules of sarcoidosis are waxy, translucent, and without scale. The malar rash of SLE may be confused with rosacea, seborrheic dermatitis, or acne.

HOW TO MAKE THE DIAGNOSIS

Punch biopsy usually confirms the diagnosis. Rarely, an additional biopsy specially processed for immunofluorescence microscopy is needed to confirm the diagnosis in patients with scarring alopecia or mucosal disease. The antinuclear antibody (ANA) is a nonspecific test. It is almost always positive in SCLE and SLE, but only in 15% to 30% of DLE patients. The anti-Ro (SS-A) antibody is frequently positive in SCLE patients; however, it should not be used to confirm or rule out the diagnosis. Antinative (double-stranded) DNA is specific for SLE, particularly renal disease.

TREATMENT

Photosensitivity is a major factor in all types of cutaneous LE. Therefore sunscreens that block UVA and UVB and sun avoidance are a cornerstone of therapy. Sunscreens must be used every day. Topical corticosteroids should be prescribed in conjunction with other agents. The strength is based on the clinical lesion and area of the body that is affected. Lesions that do not respond to topical agents can be injected intralesionally with minute amounts (less than 0.05 mL) of triamcinolone acetonide suspension in a concentration of 3 mg/mL.

Antimalarial agents are the mainstay of systemic therapy for cutaneous LE. The oral agents available include hydroxychloroquine, 200 to 400 mg daily, and chloroquine phosphate, 250 to 500 mg daily. Both agents may cause retinopathy. Ophthalmologic examination and periodic reevaluation are necessary.

CHAPTER 14

Dermatomyositis (ICD-9 710.3)

Jeffrey P. Callen, M.D.

SYMPTOMS AND SIGNS

Skin lesions of dermatomyositis (DM) are often pruritic. The characteristic lesions are the heliotrope rash and Gottron's papules. The heliotrope rash consists of a periorbital violaceous to dusky erythematous rash, which may be edematous (Fig. 14-1). Gottron's papules are erythematosus to violaceous papules or plaques found over bony prominences, particularly over the metacarpal–phalangeal joints, the proximal interphalangeal joints, and the distal interphalangeal joints (Fig. 14-2). Nail-fold changes consist of periungual telangiectasias and cuticular hypertrophy with small hemorrhagic infarcts. Patches of poikiloderma—mottled, atrophic, and telangiectatic skin—develop on exposed surfaces, such as the extensor arm and the anterior V of the neck. The scalp may be red and intensely pruritic with diffuse scale and alopecia. Calcinosis of the skin or muscle is unusual in adults but may occur in up to 40% of children with DM.

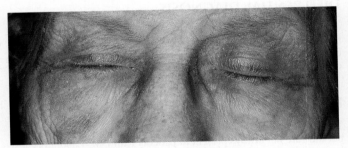

FIGURE 1. Dermatomyositis. Periorbital lilac discoloration of heliotrope rash.

More than 90% of patients with skin lesions eventually have myopathy, but the skin lesions may precede muscle disease by months to years. The myopathy of DM affects mainly the proximal muscle groups of the shoulder and pelvic girdles and is usually symmetric. Initial complaints include weakness; fatigue; inability to climb stairs, raise the arms for hair grooming or shaving; and weakness in rising from a squatting or sitting position. Arthralgias or arthritis occur in up to 25% of patients. Dysphagia is present in 20% to 50% and can be either proximal or distal. About 20% of DM patients have an associated malignancy.

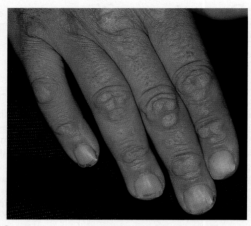

FIGURE 2. Gottron's papules are flat-topped erythematous papules and plaques over bony prominences on the dorsal hands.

DIFFERENTIAL DIAGNOSIS

The skin lesions of DM are often hard to differentiate from lupus erythematosus. Psoriasis, lichen planus, and chronic eczemas may also be considered until the classic features of DM appear. Punch biopsy can exclude all these conditions except lupus erythematosus.

HOW TO MAKE THE DIAGNOSIS

The heliotrope rash and Gottron's papules are the most helpful signs, but they are not always present in patients with DM. Laboratory testing includes serum creatine kinase or aldolase or both. An electromyogram, muscle biopsy, or MRI of the muscles may be necessary.

TREATMENT

The mainstay of therapy for myositis is systemic corticosteroids. Prednisone, 0.5 to 1 mg/kg daily by mouth, is the initial therapy. Immunosuppressive agents including methotrexate, azathioprine, cyclophosphamide, chlorambucil, or cyclosporin are used in nonresponsive patients or in patients who develop steroid-related toxicity. Low-dose methotrexate, 15 to 30 mg per week by mouth may also be effective.

Even when the myositis responds to these measures, skin disease may persist. Hydroxychloroquine, 200 to 400 mg daily by mouth, is effective treatment for skin disease in approximately 80% of patients. Finally, DM patients with cutaneous lesions are exquisitely photosensitive, so sunscreens with a sun protective factor (SPF) of at least 15 should be applied daily.

PROGNOSIS

Prognosis of patients with DM varies, depending on the series reported. Factors predisposing to poor outcome are advanced age, severe myositis, dysphagia, associated malignancy, and poor response to corticosteroid therapy.

CHAPTER 15

Urticaria (ICD-9 708.9)

Larry E. Millikan, M.D.

SYMPTOMS AND SIGNS

Urticaria is pruritic. The degree of pruritus depends on the amount of swelling. Patients often say they can watch the lesions come and go within hours. The lesions are evanescent and migratory and do not last beyond 24 hours. Urticaria presents as elevated and edematous plaques, usually pale red or pink. As the lesions spread, there is often central clearing, which leaves an arcuate or gyrate formation (Fig. 15-1).

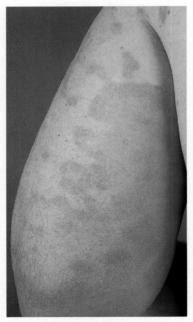

FIGURE 1. Urticaria. Central clearing of urticarial lesions leads to arcuate appearance that is sometimes confused with tinea corporis.

Urticaria may be acute or chronic. By definition, acute urticaria lasts less than 6 weeks, and chronic urticaria lasts longer. The causes of either are rarely found. Common precipitants include salicylates and penicillins. Salicylates are found in spearmint and wintergreen flavors as in toothpaste, candies, and tomatoes. Penicillins can be found in bleu cheese dressing and some dairy products. Menthol is the culprit in peppermint toothpaste or mentholated cigarettes. Other causes include foods (seafoods, strawberries, FDC Yellow #5), opiates, antibiotics, antiepileptics, and systemic diseases such as lupus erythematosus and paraproteinemias.

Urticaria can be also be caused by physical agents, such as heat, cold, ultraviolet light, and the trauma of scratching (dermatographism). Exercise-induced urticaria (cholinergic urticaria) produces small lesions 1 to 2 mm in diameter.

DIFFERENTIAL DIAGNOSIS

Erythema multiforme, urticarial vasculitis, bullous pemphigoid, and collagen vascular disease may present with widespread urticarial plaques. Atopic eczema and contact dermatitis may also be urticarial, but these are more pruritic. Miliaria and folliculitis resemble cholinergic urticaria. Urticarial lesions with central clearing resemble tinea corporis.

HOW TO MAKE THE DIAGNOSIS

Diagnosis of urticaria often can be made purely on symptoms and signs. Dermatographism can be elicited by lightly scratching the skin (Fig. 15-2). When the diagnosis is not certain, a punch biopsy may help.

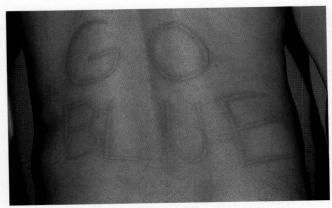

FIGURE 2. Urticaria. Dermatographism elicited after light scratching.

TREATMENT

The premise is that histamine is the major physiologic agent inducing urticaria. Since the vasculature has both H_1 and H_2 receptors, it is important to consider the use of both types of antihistamine. The caveat with most antihistamines is adequate dosing. Keep in mind that the recommended dosage is usually for a 70-kg patient. In our affluent, well-fed society, many patients are at least 50% over the average weight.

For mild, limited disease, withdrawing the causative agent may be all that is needed. In addition, oral H_1 blockers may be helpful. These include loratadine, 10 mg daily, hydroxyzine, 25 mg two to three times daily, or cyproheptadine, 4 mg four times daily. If this is not effective, an H_2 blocker, such as cimetidine, 300 mg daily by mouth, may be added. Other H_2 blockers can be effective but are more expensive. Finally, a short course of an oral corticosteroid tapered over 10 days may be needed. A good beginning dose is prednisone 1.0 mg/kg daily.

PROGNOSIS

Most patients with acute urticaria clear on therapy without discovery of a cause. The prognosis in any chronic urticaria is guarded. Patients should always understand that urticaria, acute or chronic, is a serious symptom complex that may not respond to therapy and that oral corticosteroid treatment to prevent serious airway complications may be necessary for prolonged periods of time.

CHAPTER 16
Erythema Multiforme (ICD-9 695.1)
Larry E. Millikan, M.D.

SYMPTOMS AND SIGNS

We must begin with a note on terminology. There is confusion because the term erythema multiforme (EM) describes a spectrum of disease whose boundaries seem to shift by author. Authors are either "splitters" or "lumpers."

Splitters divide the EM spectrum into several entities, beginning with mild EM and severe EM. Mild EM has mild skin involvement and sometimes mild mucosal involvement, usually the mouth. Severe EM has more advanced skin involvement and prominent mucosal involvement, including the mouth, labia, and conjunctiva. To confuse things further, some splitters label the severe form of EM the Stevens–Johnson syndrome (SJS). Furthermore, toxic epidermal necrolysis (TEN), with its massive skin sloughing, is considered in this scheme to be yet another, separate entity.

Lumpers divide the spectrum into only two groups, EM and TEN/SJS. For this book, we will use the simpler scheme of the lumpers (see Chapter 31).

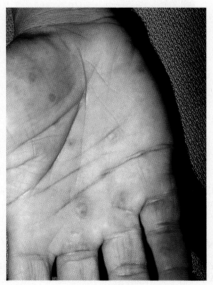

FIGURE 1. The primary sign of erythema multiforme is erythema; the classic lesion is the target.

The symptoms of EM may be minimal—a feeling of warmth or pruritus of involved skin—or severe. Bullous lesions may be very painful. Pain on the palms is a good clue to the diagnosis. The primary sign of EM is erythema; the classic lesions are targets (Fig. 16-1; see also Fig. 31-2). Target (or iris) lesions are round with a central dusky red bulls-eye surrounded by edematous concentric pink rings. EM may also be arcuate like common urticaria or bullous (Fig. 16-2). Distribution and extent of involvement can be variable. However, EM usually begins as a symmetric eruption on the extensor extremities and may progress to trunk or face involvement.

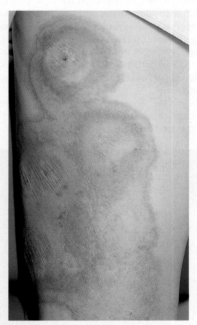

FIGURE 2. Erythema multiforme. Arcuate lesions with central clearing may resemble common urticaria.

DIFFERENTIAL DIAGNOSIS

Although the arcuate rings of urticarial lesions may be indistinguishable from EM, urticarial lesions resolve within 24 hours. Angioedema involves larger areas of skin and is indurated. Early contact dermatitis can usually be ruled out by lack of contact with an offending agent. A final consideration would be graft-versus-host disease, which occurs only in specific situations.

HOW TO MAKE THE DIAGNOSIS

The patient's history is crucial, especially when the lesions are early and there are no targets. Pain is a key symptom of EM. Check for a history of drug therapy or infection by *Mycoplasma pneumoniae* or herpes simplex. Common drugs that trigger EM are sulfonamides, penicillin, barbiturates, and phenytoin. Remember that at least 50% of EM patients have a negative history. Punch biopsy may be useful to confirm the clinical diagnosis.

TREATMENT

Elimination of a causative drug or infectious agent is most helpful for patients with EM. Pruritus can be treated with antihistamines. More advanced disease may respond to systemic oral corticosteroids such as prednisone, 1.0 mg/kg daily, in the very early phases. In TEN/SJS, the role of systemic corticosteroids is uncertain. Patients with TEN/SJS-must be treated in a burn facility.

PROGNOSIS

Mild EM in children and adults has an excellent prognosis and usually resolves within 2 to 4 weeks. Sequelae may include postinflammatory pigment changes and scarring. Suppressive treatment of herpes simplex infection may break the cycle of EM recurrence. TEN/SJS is a severe disease, which may progress to death.

CHAPTER 17

Drug Eruption (ICD-9 693.0)

Larry E. Millikan, M.D.

SYMPTOMS AND SIGNS

Symptoms of drug eruption can vary and may include itching, pruritus, burning, or frank skin pain. Symptoms usually correlate with the severity of the reaction. Skin pain is associated with severe reactions and may be a harbinger of toxic epidermal necrolysis/Stevens–Johnson syndrome (TEN/SJS). Drug reactions vary in their clinical presentation. In most cases, they occur within 3 weeks of beginning therapy. In some instances, such as penicillin eruptions in previously sensitized patients, the reaction can begin within 1 day of administration.

Urticarial and maculopapular eruptions are the most common eruptions (Fig. 17-1). Bullous reactions and erythema multiforme are less common (see Figs. 16-1 and 16-2). Fortunately, palpable purpura (cutaneous vasculitis) (see Fig. 62-1) and TEN/SJS (see Figs. 31-1, 31-2, and 31-3) are rare. Some of the more common offending drugs are peni-

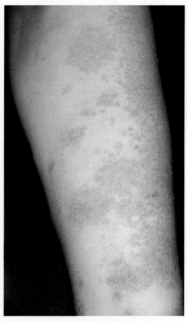

FIGURE 1. Urticarial and maculopapular eruption due to ampicillin.

48

cillins, cephalosporins, sulfonamides, phenytoin, phenobarbital, allopurinol, nonsteroidal anti-inflammatory drugs, and gold.

DIFFERENTIAL DIAGNOSIS

Erythema multiforme and TEN/SJS can be caused by other etiologies. Individual urticarial lesions disappear within 24 hours. Eczema is more pruritic, and photosensitivity reactions have the characteristic distribution on exposed skin, usually the forearms, V-area of the upper portion of the neck and the face. Viral exanthems may also be considered, although these often have accompanying respiratory or gastrointestinal symptoms.

HOW TO MAKE THE DIAGNOSIS

Diagnosis requires detective work, especially given the number of new medications introduced each year.

TREATMENT

Elimination of the suspect drug is most important. Symptomatic treatments include topical corticosteroid cream or ointment. The recommended strength depends on the degree of reaction and the patient's discomfort. Usually high-potent agents are given at first. Oral prednisone, 1 mg/kg body weight, may be needed to arrest severe reactions. Oral antihistamines may also bring relief. Some choices are cyproheptadine, 4 mg three times daily and 8 mg at night; loratidine, 10 mg daily; hydroxyzine, 10 mg three to four times daily (if patient weighs less than 50 kg) or 25 mg three to four times daily (if patient weighs over 50 kg); and cetirizine, 10 mg daily.

PROGNOSIS

Outcome is usually excellent with early treatment. TEN/SJS is a serious sign that carries significant morbidity and mortality.

CHAPTER 18

Erythema Migrans/Lyme Disease

(ICD-9 088.81)

John T. Crissey, M.D.

SYMPTOMS AND SIGNS

It is convenient to divide the course and manifestations of lyme disease (LD) into two stages: early (acute) and late (chronic).

In early LD, 80% of patients present with erythema migrans (EM). Most lesions are asymptomatic. Occasionally, the lesions burn or itch. EM is a highly characteristic skin lesion that appears first as a round or oval erythematous macule at the site of the tick bite (Fig. 18-1). A red punctum at the site of the tick attachment may be present at the center of the ring, the "bullseye" in a circular target. The incubation period is 1 to 30 days, with an average of 9 days. Any area of the skin can be affected, and lesions can be single or multiple. The lesions expand nearly 1 cm per day to reach a diameter of 10 to 30 cm. Central clearing is common, giving lesions a ringlike configuration. Regional lymphadenitis may be present. Some patients also experience several days of chills, fever, headache, fatigue, and muscle and joint pain. EM clears spontaneously in a few weeks or months.

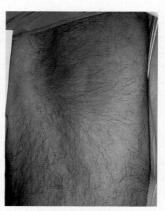

FIGURE 1. Erythema migrans. Round macule with bullseye at site of tick bite.

Late (chronic) manifestations of the infection appear weeks, months, or years after the tick bite and indicate dissemination of the infection. Intermittent arthritis affects the large joints, especially the knees. Central nervous system (CNS) involvement is common and consists of pain and weakness or numbness in arms or legs, fatigue, disturbances in vision, impaired hearing, facial paralysis (Bell's), or the signs and symptoms of meningitis—headaches, fever, stiff neck, and clouded sensorium. Cardiac involvement is less common and usually appears as a symptomatic variable atrioventricular block.

LD is caused by the spirochete, *Borrelia burgdorferi.* The organism is introduced through the bite of any of several small (2 mm) ticks of the genus *Ixodes,* which are natural parasites of deer, mice, and other mammals that inhabit forested areas (Fig. 18-2). Most cases occur in the northeastern and upper midwestern areas of the United States, as well as in northern California.

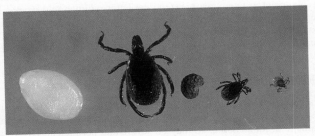

FIGURE 2. Size comparison. **Left to right:** Sesame seed, adult tick, poppy seed, nymph stage, larva stage.

DIFFERENTIAL DIAGNOSIS

Cellulitis and reactions to bites of other insects, especially spiders, can mimic EM. Multiple lesions of EM sometimes resemble erythema multiforme. Fibromyalgia, suggested by the arm and leg pains that often occur in CNS involvement in chronic LD, is the most common misdiagnosis. CNS LD can easily be mistaken for multiple sclerosis and other meningeal infections.

HOW TO MAKE THE DIAGNOSIS

The diagnosis of EM/LD is clinical. It is based on a history of exposure to an area where Lyme disease is endemic and on the presence of EM. The causative organism can be identified in situ in punch biopsy material taken from EM lesions. It can also be cultured on special media unavailable in most places. Neither method is practical. Two serologic tests for antibodies to *B. burgdorferi* are available, the ELISA assay and Western immunoblot. Results are often negative in early LD, but are more useful in the later stages. The consensus is that both test results must be positive to establish a diagnosis by serologic means. Better tests are being developed.

TREATMENT

Antibiotic choice and dosage schedules are in a state of flux at present. Health care providers are encouraged to consult the latest literature for the latest developments. For now, doxycycline, tetracycline, amoxicillin, penicillin G, cefuroxime axetil, ceftriaxone, and cefotaximine all are active against *B. burgdorferi*. For early LD, use doxycycline, 100 mg twice daily by mouth for 21 days (amoxicillin, 25 to 50 mg/kg daily for children under 8 years). For arthritis and mild cardiovascular involvement in later stages, extend the latter regimen to 4 weeks. Patients with neurologic involvement are treated with intravenous ceftriaxone sodium, 2 g daily for 14 to 28 days. No current data support the treatment of patients with asymptomatic tick bites from endemic areas.

PROGNOSIS

The outlook for cure in acute LD is uniformly good. Late cases usually respond well, although some are refractory and require retreatment. Damage to joints and CNS may be severe and permanent. Deaths are rare.

CHAPTER 19

Candidosis (ICD-9 112.9)

Lawrence Charles Parish, M.D.

SYMPTOMS AND SIGNS

Candida infection on the skin can be asymptomatic or pruritic and burning. Previously called monilial dermatitis, it is a yeast infection, most often caused by Candida albicans, an organism that is a frequent inhabitant of the gut and the vagina. Candidosis is characterized by red papules and macules that may become confluent, leaving isolated or "satellite" papules and macules at the periphery (Fig. 19-1). Occasionally, the areas become raw, eroded, and oozing. It is often found in the intertriginous areas such as the groin, on the perianal region, and under the breasts, particularly in obese patients. *Candida* balanitis and *Candida* vulvovaginitis often pingpong between partners. The history often reveals that the patient had diarrhea several days before the onset of the dermatitis or that the female partner has had a vaginal discharge. Diabetics are predisposed to candidosis, and the condition can be florid in immunocompromised patients.

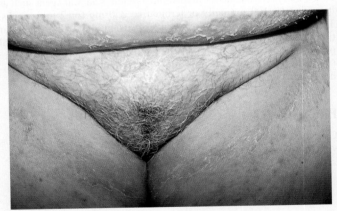

FIGURE 1. Candidosis. Erythema, scaling, and satellite lesions in the groin.

Special types of candidosis include oral candidosis or thrush, in which there are white papules or patches inside the mouth or on the tongue. **Pseudoblastomyces interdigitale** presents as red, scaling areas between the fingers, often under a ring. Monilial paronychia causes redness, induration, swelling, and tenderness around the nail.

DIFFERENTIAL DIAGNOSIS

Seborrheic dermatitis may be confused with candidosis, but the lack of satellite lesions points toward the former. Also, seborrheic dermatitis is found in more locations including the scalp, glabella, paranasal area, submentum, sternum, axillae, umbilicus, and groin. Contact dermatitis might not be symmetric, and the satellite lesions would be missing. A dermatophyte infection might show central clearing and more scaling.

HOW TO MAKE THE DIAGNOSIS

Candidosis is diagnosed by clinical inspection. A positive 10% potassium hydroxide scraping or culture on fungal medium confirms the diagnosis.

TREATMENT

Localized areas on the skin lend themselves to topical treatment with antifungal creams of the imidazole or allylamine classes applied daily or twice daily—depending on the agent—for 2 to 3 weeks (see Table 23-1). Extensive cutaneous involvement requires an oral agent such as itraconazole, 100 mg daily or terbinafine 250 mg for 2 to 4 weeks. Thrush can be treated with nystatin suspension, 100,000 U/mL four times daily, or clotrimazole trouche, 10 mg five times daily. Monilial paronychia is treated systemically with itraconazole or terbinafine (same doses as above), or topically with thymol 4% in absolute alcohol applied four times daily.

PROGNOSIS

Candidosis can be prevented by keeping the areas dry, treating the vulvovaginitis, and keeping the diabetes under control.

CHAPTER 20

Psoriasis (ICD-9 696.1)

James C. Shaw, M.D.

SYMPTOMS AND SIGNS

Psoriasis is usually asymptomatic, although some patients can have pruritus that is sometimes severe. The disease affects 1% of the population of the United States. It usually begins by age 10 years, although patients may present any time later. The cardinal features of psoriasis are sharply circumscribed, thick plaques of erythematous skin covered with silvery scales (Fig. 20-1). Nail involvement is common and can be the key to diagnosis. Look for pitting and nail plate dystrophy (Fig. 20-2). The isomorphic (Koebner's) phenomenon can be a clue to diagnosis. This consists of the development of psoriatic skin changes after physical trauma to the skin, such as local abrasions or sunburn. Several types of psoriasis exist.

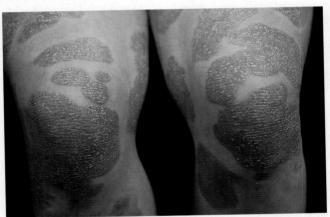

FIGURE 1. Plaque psoriasis is sharply demarcated from surrounding normal skin.

Plaque psoriasis presents as thick, fixed plaques on the extensor elbows, knees, scalp, lower back, sacral area, and scalp. Demarcation between normal and psoriatic skin is sharp. Any area of the body can be affected, but the face is usually spared. One variant, called **inverse psoriasis** affects intertriginous areas of the groin, intergluteal cleft, axillae, and inframammary areas.

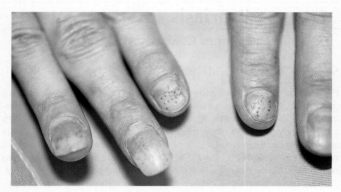

FIGURE 2. Psoriatic nail pitting with nail plate dystrophy.

Guttate psoriasis appears as multiple 0.5- to 1.0-cm psoriatic papules, which develop abruptly on the trunk and extremities, frequently associated with a recent streptococcal pharyngitis (Fig. 20-3).

In pustular psoriasis, multiple superficial pustules that may coalesce into pustular lakes develop on previously normal skin or on top of typical, preexisting psoriatic plaques. Pustules are usually all over the body, but a variant of pustular psoriasis is limited to the palms and soles.

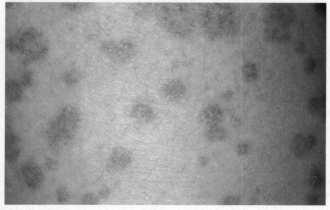

FIGURE 3. Guttate psoriasis is associated with streptococcal pharyngitis.

A rare presentation of psoriasis is a total body erythroderma. This can be life-threatening owing to fluid and electrolyte disturbances and thermal dysregulation.

Psoriasis in HIV-infected individuals is often severe. It commonly has features of both pustular psoriasis and Reiter's syndrome.

Psoriatic arthritis can be present in up to 30% of psoriatics. It usually develops by age 30 to 40 years and commonly affects the fingers (polyarticular type) or knees, ankles, and metatarsal-phalangeal joints (oligoarticular type). Severity of joint disease does not necessarily correlate with severity of the skin disease.

Several drugs can exacerbate psoriasis, including beta blockers, angiotensin converting enzyme inhibitors, calcium channel blockers, and antimalarials.

DIFFERENTIAL DIAGNOSIS

All papulosquamous diseases are included in the differential diagnosis. Pityriasis rosea can resemble guttate psoriasis but the herald patch and Christmas tree distribution are distinguishing. In discoid lupus erythematosus, thick plaques look like psoriasis, and biopsy may be required to make the distinction. In subacute cutaneous lupus erythematosus, plaques are usually thinner than in typical psoriasis. Unlike psoriasis, both forms of cutaneous lupus are exacerbated by sunlight and often appear on sun-exposed skin. Lichen planus is violaceous and less scaling.

HOW TO MAKE THE DIAGNOSIS

Correct diagnosis of psoriasis is usually made by physical examination. Punch biopsy can be diagnostic in difficult cases. Careful examination of scalp, umbilicus, intergluteal cleft, and nails and evidence of Koebner's phenomenon can provide clues.

TREATMENT

For limited disease (less than 20% of the body), emollient creams and ointments, and moderate to super-potent topical corticosteroid ointments and creams are the mainstay of therapy. Because psoriasis is a chronic condition, the strength of topical corticosteroid should be reduced as soon as possible to avoid side effects. Addition of crude coal tar 2% to 5% into the topical corticosteroid can be helpful. (The pharmacist will do the compounding.) Calcipotriene 0.005% cream or solution twice daily and the topical retinoid tazarotene gel 0.05% to 0.1% once daily are alternatives to topical corticosteroids.

For moderate disease (greater than 20% percent of the body), topical therapies are more difficult to use. Ultraviolet (UV) light treatments either with UVB or the combination of UVA plus oral psoralens (PUVA) are frequently effective.

Widespread disease, pustular psoriasis, and severe psoriatic arthritis require systemic therapies. Methotrexate, systemic retinoid (acetretin), and cyclosporin A are used alone or in combination.

PROGNOSIS

Psoriasis is usually a lifelong disease. Patients may enjoy periods of improvement, but most rely on maintenance treatment to control disease. Morbidity can be significant in patients with psoriatic arthritis and pustular forms. In most cases, there are no medical complications.

CHAPTER 21

Pityriasis Rosea (ICD-9 696.3)

Larry E. Millikan, M.D.

SYMPTOMS AND SIGNS

Pruritus in pityriasis rosea (PR) is usually absent or mild. Rarely is it severe in the papular form of the disease. Many patients recall a "herald patch" as the first sign of PR. The herald patch is red, scaling, and often on the trunk, measuring up to 6 to 7 cm in diameter (Fig. 21-1). Up to 3 weeks later, smaller ovoid macules, 1 to 3 cm in diameter, appear on the trunk and proximal extremities. These lesions sometimes follow a dermatomal distribution on the back, giving the famous "Christmas tree" pattern of PR. But this pattern is not always present. It is far more useful to find lesions with a central collarette of scale, which is a more reliable finding that can make the diagnosis (Fig. 21-2). A rare inverse form of PR causes lesions on the palms, soles, and face.

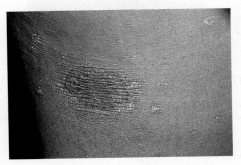

FIGURE 1. Pityriasis rosea. The herald patch is easily confused with psoriasis or eczema.

DIFFERENTIAL DIAGNOSIS

Patients with secondary syphilis have lymphadenopathy. Tinea corporis, psoriasis, and eczema are other considerations, especially when there is a herald patch. In tinea, microscopic examination of scales will show hyphae. Psoriatic lesions, more scaling, and the typical distribution of knees, elbows, nails, and scalp are unlike PR. Eczema is far more pruritic.

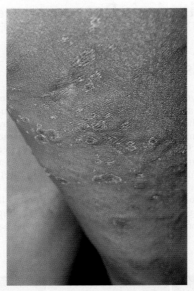

FIGURE 2. Pityriasis rosea. The same patient with typical ovoid lesions showing collarettes of scale.

HOW TO MAKE THE DIAGNOSIS

Diagnosis of PR is clinical, based on history, herald patch followed by typical lesions and distribution, and general well-being of the patient.

TREATMENT

Treatment of PR depends on symptoms but is frequently not necessary. Low-potent topical corticosteroid ointment or cream can reduce itch. Another approach is compounding 1/4% to 1/2% menthol—with or without 1/4% to 1/2% phenol—in moisturizing lotion or cream. Ultraviolet light from the sun is helpful early in the course of disease.

PROGNOSIS

PR is a benign condition and resolves in 2 to 3 months. It recurs in about 10% of patients.

CHAPTER 22
Lichen Planus (ICD-9 697.0)
Larry E. Millikan, M.D.

SYMPTOMS AND SIGNS

Lichen planus (LP) can be very pruritic. The classic signs are scaling and purple-to-brown polygonal papules on the wrists, forearms, and legs (Fig. 22-1). Papules are flat on top. A white, shiny lacy pattern,

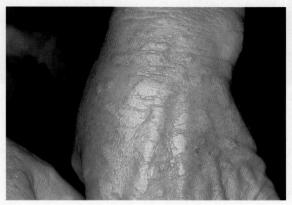

FIGURE 1. Lichen planus. Flat-topped, purple, polygonal papules with shiny, lacy pattern of Wickham's striae.

called Wickham's striae, can sometimes be seen on the surface of the papules after application of a drop of oil. A hand lens may be needed to detect this. About two thirds of LP patients have reticular, white patches or plaques on the buccal mucosa (Fig. 22-2). The head of the penis may also be affected. Hypertrophic LP is a variant, in which thick, large plaques appear on the distal extremities, particularly on the shins. LP of the nails may cause obliteration of the nail fold (pterygium), longitudinal ridging, and pitting.

DIFFERENTIAL DIAGNOSIS

Few other papulosquamous disorders are as pruritic as LP. Guttate psoriasis usually has other lesions that are classic for psoriasis and never has Wickham's striae or mouth lesions. Lichenoid drug eruptions can mimic LP; lesions due to drugs may be identical clinically and histologically. Drugs most likely to cause an LP-like eruption are gold, chloroquine, quinacrine, quinine, tetracycline, griseofulvin, dapsone, penicillamine, and beta blockers.

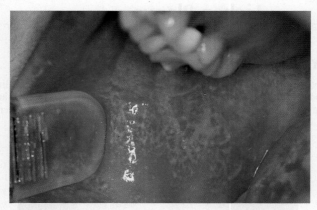

FIGURE 2. Lichen planus. White, reticular pattern on the buccal mucosa is often a key to the diagnosis.

Patients with very limited early forms of tinea corporis may present with perifollicular papules, but these papules are rarely pruritic and hyphae can be found by microscope examination of scales.

HOW TO MAKE THE DIAGNOSIS

Diagnosis of LP is established by careful examination. Lesions on the buccal mucosa are helpful. Patients should be tested for hepatitis C, since LP has been associated with this infection. The history may reveal offending drugs. Punch biopsy of a typical lesion usually confirms the diagnosis.

THERAPY

Therapy for LP often requires trial of different agents. High-potent or super-potent topical corticosteroid ointments or creams seem to be the most consistently effective treatment. Longstanding extensive LP may respond to retinoids or dapsone. Mucous membrane lesions may be treated with potent topical corticosteroids or intralesional injections of triamcinolone acetonide suspension in concentrations of 2.5 to 10 mg/mL to a maximum of 10 to 15 mg weekly.

PROGNOSIS

Most patients with LP heal within 1 year, often with some degree of postinflammatory hyperpigmentation. Recurrences occur in less than 50% of patients.

CHAPTER 23

Tinea (ICD-9 110.0 capitis; 110.2 manuum; 110.3 cruris; 110.4 pedis; 110.5 corporis)

Lawrence Charles Parish, M.D.

SYMPTOMS AND SIGNS

Superficial fungal infections may be asymptomatic, pruritic, or burning. They are often to referred to as "ringworm" because the characteristic lesion is a round, scaling, red area with central clearing and sharp, elevated borders. Most dermatophyte infections are caused by species of *Trichophyton*, *Epidermophyton*, or *Microsporon*. The infections are described by location.

Tinea corporis can involve any part of the body. The lesions are oval to round, red, and scaling patches with a central area of clearing (Fig. 23-1). The patterns can be polycyclic. **Tinea cruris**, or jock itch,

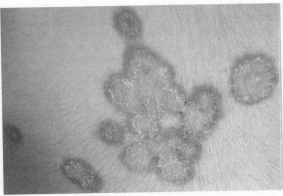

FIGURE 1. Tinea corporis due to *Microsporon canis* showing red rings with peripheral scale and central clearing.

appears as diffuse redness and scaling with sharp borders. **Tinea pedis**, or athlete's foot, appears in three forms. The most common, "moccasin foot," presents as scaling on the soles, sometimes with erythema and crusting. Intertriginous infection manifests as fissuring and scaling between the toes—usually the fourth and fifth toes. Inflammatory and vesicular infection occurs on the instep and sole. Moccasin foot often appears along with **tinea manuum**, in which the "two-feet-one-hand" pattern is common and is a clue to diagnosis (Fig. 23-2).

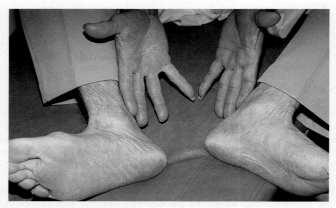

FIGURE 2. Dermatophyte infection with two-feet-one-hand pattern; right hand infected.

Tinea capitis is generally limited to children. Tinea tonsurans causes the so-called "black dot" type of tinea capitis, in which broken hairs appear as dark spots on the scalp. When the infection is caused by *M. canis*, there are scaling and well-defined patches of hair loss with broken hairs. With more inflammation and infection, a red boggy area, a kerion, may develop.

DIFFERENTIAL DIAGNOSIS

Tinea corporis may be confused with contact dermatitis or atopic dermatitis, as can tinea cruris and tinea pedis. Jock itch can mimic intertrigo due to tight underwear. Tinea pedis can mimic psoriasis. Tinea capitis is sometimes confused with alopecia areata or seborrheic dermatitis. Tinea faciei is often mistaken for eczema.

HOW TO MAKE THE DIAGNOSIS

Clinical inspection is generally sufficient to make the diagnosis, but 10% potassium hydroxide scrapings showing branching hyphae or positive fungal cultures confirm the clinical impression (Fig. 23-3). The Wood's light examination for tinea capitis is only rarely helpful today because the causative agents are endothritic and do not fluoresce; however, *M. audouinii* and *M. canis* do fluoresce. Examination of plucked hairs and surrounding scalp scales often reveals organisms under the microscope.

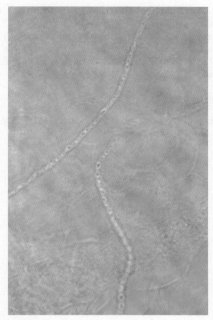

FIGURE 3. Hyphae diagnostic of dermatophyte infection (10% potassium hydroxide)

TREATMENT

Fungal infections of the skin itself can be treated with topical antifungal creams of the imidazole or allylamines classes (Table 23-1). With

TABLE 23–1. *Antifungal Creams*

Class	Schedule	Brand
Imidazoles		
Clotrimazole 1%	Twice daily	Generic available
Econazole 1%	Once daily	Spectazole[a]
Ketoconazole 2%	Once daily	Nizoral
Miconazole 2%	Twice daily	Generic available
Oxiconazole 1%	Once daily	Oxistat
Allylamines		
Naftidine 1%	Once daily	Naftin
Terbinafine 1%	Twice daily	Lamisil

[a] Should be used twice daily for *Candida* infection.

65

more extensive or chronic involvement, oral agents such as terbinafine 250 mg are taken daily for 3 to 4 weeks.

Tinea capitis requires oral griseofulvin (microsize), 10 to 15 mg/kg daily for at least 6 weeks, or terbinafine, 250 mg daily for 2 to 4 weeks. Absorption of griseofulvin increases if taken with fatty foods.

PROGNOSIS

Superficial fungal infections are readily cured with proper treatment.

CHAPTER 24

Tinea Versicolor (ICD-9 111.0)

Lawrence Charles Parish, M.D.

SIGNS AND SYMPTOMS

Patients with tinea versicolor (TV) may complain of mild pruritus. Because the organism, *Malassezia furfur*, needs a warm, moist area high in lipids, TV often occurs in the warmer months or during the winter among patients who engage in vigorous exercise with sweating. TV generally does not appear before puberty. It is characterized by sharply demarcated hyperpigmented or hypopigmented scaling patches on the trunk, neck, and proximal arms (Fig. 24-1). It is called "versicolor" because the coloring can be whitish, brownish, or even reddish, depending on the normal color of the patient's skin. The lesions give a fine, branlike scale with minimal scratching. Patients are often not aware of the condition until they are suntanned and the hypopigmentations caused by TV is more noticeable.

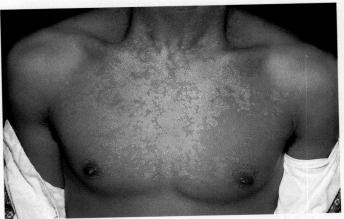

FIGURE 1. Tinea versicolor. Sharply demarcated hyper- and hypopigmented patches on the trunk.

DIFFERENTIAL DIAGNOSIS

Because the scaling is mild, TV can be confused with a drug eruption, neurodermatitis, or psoriasis, especially guttate psoriasis. If scaling is minimal, the hypopigmented patches can resemble vitiligo.

HOW TO MAKE THE DIAGNOSIS

Examination of scales under the microscope using potassium hydroxide shows the characteristic hyphae and budding—"spaghetti and meatballs"—of TV (Fig. 24-2). The areas fluoresce green with a Wood's light.

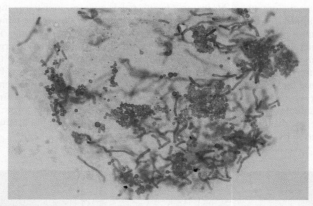

FIGURE 2. "Spaghetti and meatballs" of tinea versicolor (10% potassium hydroxide with Parker ink).

TREATMENT

There are many treatment regimens for TV. Antifungal creams of the imidazole or allylamines classes all are effective (see Table 23-1). Remember that up to 10 g of cream is needed for each daily treatment. An older regimen is selenium sulfide shampoo, 2.5% daily for at least 2 weeks. Oral antifungals, such as terbinafine 250 mg daily for 7 to 10 days, recently have been recommended as effective.

PROGNOSIS

Scaling disappears in a few weeks, but pigmentation does not return to normal for several months. Unfortunately, although TV can be treated very effectively, it cannot be cured. Recurrences can occur annually for up to 20 years. Patients should be warned to expect recurrence in summer months or during the winter if they are devoted gym goers.

CHAPTER 25

Secondary Syphilis (ICD-9 091.3)

John T. Crissey, M.D.

SYMPTOMS AND SIGNS

The lesions of secondary syphilis (SS) are discrete asymptomatic, ery-thematous to copper-colored, macular, and maculopapular lesions, which present on the trunk and genitalia. A prodrome of sore throat and flu-like symptoms may precede the lesions by a few days. The face is usually heavily involved, especially in the seborrheic areas and along the hair line. Brownish or coppery macules and slightly scaly papules often appear on palms and soles (Fig. 25-1). More than any other fea-ture, these lesions should alert the examiner to the possibility of syphilis.

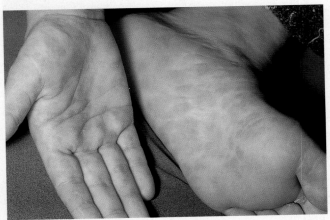

FIGURE 1. Secondary syphilis. Copper-colored macular lesions on palms and soles.

In other cases, SS lesions have a pronounced tendency to assume an-nular configurations, particularly in black patients. Face, anogenital ar-eas, palms and soles, axillae, and periumbilical areas may be involved. Because of their size and configuration, these lesions are often called "nickel and dime syphilids" (Fig. 25-2). Mucous membrane lesions in-clude a transient diffuse redness of the throat and the so-called mucous patches. The latter are slightly elevated round or oval papules, 5 to 12 mm in diameter, faintly inflammatory and covered with a pearly or grayish membrane. Lesions at the labial commissures may take the

69

form of "split" or fissured papules, easily confused with ordinary per-lèche. Mucocutaneous lesions in the genitalia and anal areas may appear as condylomata lata, which vary in morphology from slightly pedunculated, flat papules to smooth and button-like lesions or large cauliflower-like vegetations.

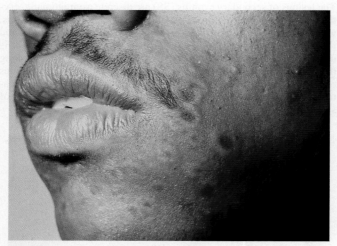

FIGURE 2. Secondary syphilis. Nickel and dime syphilid commonly presents on the face.

Other signs include more or less generalized nontender, rubbery lymphadenopathy, which occurs in about 85% of cases, and a non-scarring patchy or "moth-eaten" scalp alopecia.

Syphilis in patients infected with HIV presents special problems. Atypical clinical presentations are common, particularly ulcerating secondary lesions and pronounced systemic symptoms—the so-called "malignant syphilis." Central nervous system (CNS) involvement is unusually common—16% to 40% in some studies.

DIFFERENTIAL DIAGNOSIS

Guttate psoriasis, pityriasis rosea, and widespread lichen planus sometimes resemble SS. The absence of other signs of SS help to establish the proper diagnosis.

HOW TO MAKE THE DIAGNOSIS

Syphilis is a laboratory diagnosis. The standard nontreponemal sero-logic test, the rapid plasma reagin (RPR), is positive in almost all cases of SS. To rule out false-positive reactions, a positive RPR should be confirmed by a treponemal test such as the MHA-TP before instituting treatment.

TREATMENT

SS can be treated successfully with intramuscular benzathine penicillin G, 2.4 million units once weekly for 2 weeks. Penicillin-allergic pa-tients may be treated with oral tetracycline, 500 mg four times daily for 15 days. After treatment, titered RPR should be performed every 3 to 6 months for 2 years to rule out relapse or reinfection. In the presence of HIV infection, nontreponemal serologic tests are unreliable guides to treatment response, and conventional treatment schedules appear to be inadequate. Current literature should be consulted for the latest in the proper management of these difficult cases.

PROGNOSIS

Response to treatment in otherwise normal patients is excellent. Prog-nosis in patients with AIDS is guarded.

CHAPTER 26
Bullous Pemphigoid (ICD-9 694.4)
Jeffrey P. Callen, M.D.

SYMPTOMS AND SIGNS

Bullous pemphigoid (BP) is often pruritic. Patients are usually over 60 years of age and present with tense bullae on normal skin (Fig. 26-1) or on an urticarial lesion. The bullae are subepidermal and eventually break, leaving an erosion. Healing occurs with temporary dyspigmentation, but without scarring. Mucous membranes are rarely affected in BP. However, a variant known as benign mucous membrane pemphigoid (cicatricial pemphigoid) affects primarily the mucosal surfaces, most often the mouth and eyes, and can result in blindness. BP may be caused by thiazide diuretics, spironolactone, furosemide, captopril, penicillamine, phenothiazines, tricyclic antidepressants, or benzodiazepines. BP is not a marker for internal malignancy as previously believed.

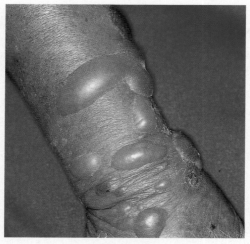

FIGURE 1. Bullous pemphigoid. Tense bullae on normal-appearing skin.

DIFFERENTIAL DIAGNOSIS

Bullous impetigo may look like BP, although it is primarily in inter-triginous areas and impetigo bullae are flaccid. Other rare, subepidermal blistering disorders must be considered because therapy often differs.

These include linear immunoglobulin A (IgA) disease, dermatitis herpetiformis, and epidermolysis bullosa acquisita. In patients without blisters, the differential diagnosis includes urticaria and insect bite reactions.

HOW TO MAKE THE DIAGNOSIS

Punch biopsies should include both an intact blister for routine processing and a biopsy of adjacent normal-appearing skin for immunofluorescence microscopy. These must be sent in Michel's transport media to a laboratory accustomed to performing these studies. BP is characterized by the deposition of IgG in the lamina lucida part of the basement membrane. Serum for indirect immunofluorescence, looking for circulating anti–basement membrane antibodies, should be also be sent to a reliable laboratory. Results of serum tests vary from one laboratory to the next. Thus, the selection of an appropriate consultant is critical. Results that do not fit with the clinical diagnosis should be repeated.

TREATMENT

Patients with BP vary in symptomatology. This factor as well as their age and preexisting medical conditions should be considered when making a decision about therapy. Drugs that cause BP should be discontinued. Oral corticosteroids such as prednisone, 1 to 2 mg/kg daily, are almost always effective. However, in this population steroids frequently result in toxicity. Oral niacinamide, 500 mg three times daily, plus tetracycline, 500 mg three times daily, is sometimes a worthy alternative. Many patients are given immunosuppressive or cytotoxic agents for their steroid-sparing effect. Methotrexate, azathioprine, and cyclosporin are among the favored choices.

PROGNOSIS

BP rarely threatens life. Control results in less risk of secondary infection that may complicate eroded skin. Often, the disease burns out in 3 to 5 years.

CHAPTER 27
Impetigo (ICD-9 684)
James C. Shaw, M.D.

SYMPTOMS AND SIGNS

Impetigo is usually asymptomatic or mildly symptomatic. It begins as one or more red papules and over 2 to 3 days expands to a crusted patch. The condition can be nonbullous or bullous. In nonbullous impetigo, there are circular patches of scaling, superficial erosions, and honey-colored crusts (Fig. 27-1). The patches are usually periorificial on the face, especially around the nose and mouth. Bullous impetigo presents as flaccid, pus-filled lakes, which are often eroded at the time of presentation. Impetigo occurs most commonly in intertriginous areas (Fig. 27-2). Bullae are 1 cm to 3 cm in diameter. There are no constitutional symptoms. Children are affected most often, although impetigo is not rare in adolescents and adults.

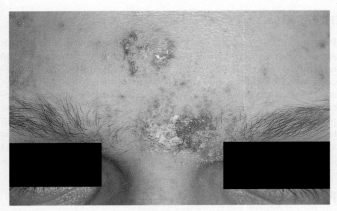

FIGURE 1. Nonbullous impetigo with scaling, superficial erosions, and honey-colored crusts.

DIFFERENTIAL DIAGNOSIS

Tinea faciale has a similar appearance on the face but is usually more pruritic and is not typically periorificial. Tinea faciale can be anywhere on the face. Herpes zoster vesicles are unilateral or dermatomal. Herpes simplex must also be considered.

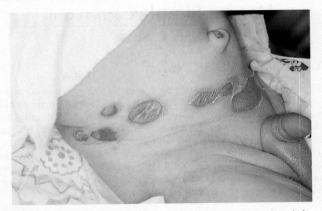

FIGURE 2. Bullous impetigo with flaccid, pus-filled bullae and eroded areas.

HOW TO MAKE THE DIAGNOSIS

Examination is usually sufficient to make the diagnosis of impetigo. The typical 2- to 3-day onset also helps make the diagnosis. A bacterial culture for group A β-hemolytic streptococci or *Staphylococcus aureus* can be taken to confirm the diagnosis. The specimen should be taken from the base of the lesion.

TREATMENT

The mainstay of treatment for impetigo is systemic antibiotics that cover both the streptococci and the staphylococci involved. Good choices for adults are dicloxacillin, 250 mg four times daily, or cephalexin, 250 mg four times daily by mouth. For penicillin-allergic patients, oral erythromycin, 250 mg four times daily, can be used. Dosages for children must calculated by body weight. Mupirocin ointment 2% four times daily has been used successfully as single-drug therapy in mild cases. It can be initiated while awaiting culture results and sensitivities.

PROGNOSIS

Impetigo is highly contagious until therapy is started. Complete recovery is the norm and requires up to 2 weeks of treatment. Scarring is rare. Glomerulonephritis is an unusual complication of impetigo after infection with certain strains of *Streptococcus*.

CHAPTER 28

Herpes Simplex (ICD-9 054.9)

James C. Shaw

SYMPTOMS AND SIGNS

Patients with primary herpes simplex virus (HSV) infection complain of burning and pain in the involved area and malaise or low-grade fever. One or two days later, lesions appear. Recurrent HSV causes tingling, burning, or itching one day before the lesions appear. HSV can cause erosive disease in patients who are immunosuppressed.

HSV type 1 commonly infects nongenital skin, usually the face and most often the lips or mouth. Oral HSV presents as multiple shallow ulcerations in the mouth or grouped clear vesicles on the vermilion border of the lip. Impetiginization is common (Fig. 28-1).

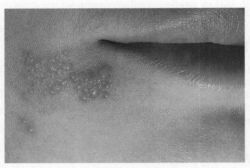

FIGURE 1. HSV 1 most commonly affects the face and mouth.

HSV type 2 usually infects anogenital skin. It appears as grouped vesicles or papules, 1 mm to 4 mm in diameter on a red base (Fig. 28-2). Usually, there are five to ten lesions in the group. There may be considerable edema. Most individuals with HSV 2 do not present with a primary infection, but with a first recurrence.

HSV may also infect by inoculation, causing herpetic whitlow on the fingers. This condition is seen most often in health care workers, particularly dentists, dental technicians, and anesthesiologists.

DIFFERENTIAL DIAGNOSIS

Patients with tinea faciale complain of more pruritus than HSV patients and have deeper papules and erythema, and no vesicles. Im-

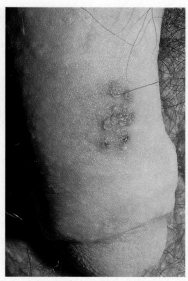

FIGURE 2. HSV 2. Clear vesicles with superficial erosions on the penis.

petigo has honey-colored crusts and pus. Herpes zoster lesions appear in many clusters and are dermatomal. Aphthous ulcers are usually singular.

HOW TO MAKE THE DIAGNOSIS

HSV is often diagnosed clinically, but a positive Tzanck preparation, done in the office laboratory, confirms the diagnosis. First, unroof a vesicle and gently smear scrapings from the base onto a glass microscope slide. Next, fix the specimen lightly with heat or absolute alcohol. Then, stain it for 2 minutes with 5% methylene blue or Wright–Giemsa stain. Finally, observe under the microscope large, multinucleated keratinocytes (Fig. 28-3). Findings are identical with those of herpes simplex and herpes zoster. The direct fluorescent antibody test can distinguish between the two viruses; obtain a smear as for a Tzanck preparation and send for processing in the hospital laboratory. Results can be obtained within hours. Viral culture, if positive, takes 1 to 3 days.

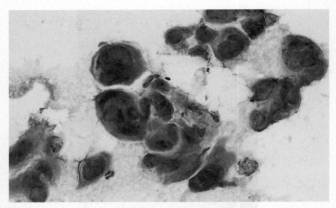

FIGURE 3. Tzanck preparation reveals multinucleated, giant keratinocytes in both herpes simplex and herpes zoster infections (methylene blue).

TREATMENT

Treat early with oral agents to stop viral replication. After several days, the cellular damage has occurred and antiviral therapy may not help. For acute HSV, whether primary or recurrent, use oral acyclovir, 200 mg five times daily for 5 days, or valacyclovir, 1,000 mg twice daily for 5 days. Oral famciclovir, 125 mg twice daily for 5 days, may also be used for acute disease. For chronic suppressive therapy, acyclovir, 400 mg two or three times daily, is often effective.

PROGNOSIS

Because HSV is contagious, patients should avoid close contact with others during the acute phase until lesions are complete healed. Genital herpes infection in pregnant women can infect the baby perinatally, and patients should alert their obstetrician if they have any symptoms or signs of active genital HSV infection.

CHAPTER 29

Herpes Zoster (ICD-9 053.9)

James C. Shaw, M.D

SYMPTOMS AND SIGNS

Herpes zoster usually begins with a 1- to 2-day prodrome of pain or burning in a dermatomal distribution. The discomfort of zoster is deep like a neuralgia or superficial on the skin. Pain can be severe. In chest or abdominal locations, prodromal pain can mimic cardiac, musculoskeletal, or intraperitoneal diseases.

The eruption consists of red papules or clear vesicles on a red base. The lesions, 2 to 4 mm in diameter, can be individual or grouped and are in a dermatomal distribution (Fig. 29-1). They often progress to confluent vesicles, which then erode and crust over. Secondary bacterial infection is common. Older patients are more likely to develop extensive involvement and severe pain. In severe cases and in immunocompromised patients, more than a single dermatome can be affected.

Herpes zoster is caused by reactivation of varicella-zoster infection (chickenpox), usually suffered years before.

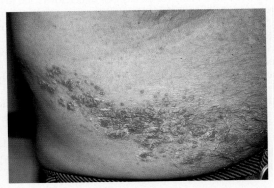

FIGURE 1. Herpes zoster. Typical dermatomal distribution on the trunk.

DIFFERENTIAL DIAGNOSIS

Herpes simplex recurrences are dermatomal, but typically appear on the lip or genitals. Insect bites, folliculitis, and tinea capitis can look the same as herpes zoster on the scalp. Cellulitis and erysipelas have considerable edema and erythema, especially when they affect the face. Human immunodeficiency virus (HIV) infection should be considered in all patients with herpes zoster.

HOW TO MAKE THE DIAGNOSIS

Herpes zoster is often a clinical diagnosis. Some laboratory measures may help. Tzanck smear (see Fig. 28-3) and punch biopsy cannot differentiate herpes zoster from primary herpes simplex virus (HSV) infection. Viral cultures of zoster are more often negative than positive and require up to 21 days for results. Moreover, if erosions and crusts have formed or if the lesions are drying, chances of a positive culture are even lower. Direct fluorescent antibody test, however, can distinguish herpes zoster from HSV within several hours. The test is done by the laboratory on a smear obtained in the same manner as for the Tzanck test.

TREATMENT

Because herpes zoster is self-limited, treatment is based on severity. Early treatment reduces the incidence and degree of postherpetic neuralgia. The dose of oral acyclovir for immunocompetent patients is 800 mg five times daily for 5 to 7 days. An alternative is valacyclovir, 1,000 mg three times daily for 10 days, or famciclovir, 500 mg or 750 mg three times daily for 7 days. For immunosuppressed patients, acyclovir 500 mg/m^2 body surface area is given intravenously every 8 hours for 10 days.

For immunocompetent patients, adjunct systemic corticosteroids may reduce lesion healing time, acute neuritis, and the need for narcotic analgesia. One regimen is oral prednisone, 60 mg daily for 1 week followed by 30 mg daily for a second week.

Postherpetic neuralgia may require treatment with narcotic analgesics or tricyclic antidepressants such as amitriptyline 50 mg to 100 mg daily by mouth.

Oral antibacterial antibiotics are needed only if there is evidence of secondary infection: dicloxacillin, cephalexin, or erythromycin, 250 mg four times daily are equally effective.

PROGNOSIS

Most cases of herpes zoster resolve with only mild scarring. Involvement of the tip of the nose is an important sign of potential corneal or conjunctival involvement because of involvement of the ophthalmic branch of the trigeminal nerve, and ophthalmologic consultation is warranted. Ramsay Hunt syndrome may occur when there is involvement of the geniculate ganglion. Recurrences are uncommon because immunity is boosted by an episode of herpes zoster. Postherpetic neuralgia is common in geriatric patients with severe disease. Immunocompromised patients can experience severe local or disseminated disease.

Herpes zoster is contagious to those who have not had varicella. Transmission is by direct contact with lesions.

CHAPTER 30

Pemphigus Vulgaris (ICD-9 694.5)

Jeffrey P. Callen, M.D.

SYMPTOMS AND SIGNS

Pemphigus is a blistering disease of the skin and mucous membranes. There are at least two major variants: pemphigus vulgaris (PV) and pemphigus foliaceus (PF). Most patients are between ages 40 and 60. PV patients often present with painful oral ulcers (Fig. 30-1). The mouth sores or desquamative gingivitis are followed by skin lesions including flaccid bullae, which may be so fragile that they are sometimes not observed, and only erosions and crusts are seen (Fig. 30-2). Oral PV can develop by itself in the absence of skin disease. In contrast, the lesions of PF are superficial, are localized to the head, neck, and upper trunk, and rarely involve the mouth.

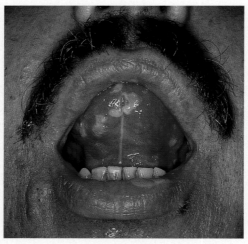

FIGURE 1. Pemphigus vulgaris. Painful ulcerations in the mouth.

DIFFERENTIAL DIAGNOSIS

Impetigo and impetiginized eczema have typical honey-colored crusts. Seborrheic dermatitis is scaling. Bullous pemphigoid lesions are tense and not flaccid, and oral disease is rare. Aphthous stomatitis lesions are punched out. Patients with erosive oral lichen planus usually have typ-

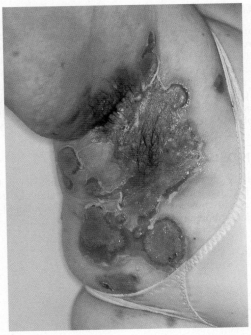

FIGURE 2. Pemphigus vulgaris. Severe erosions and crusts in the axilla.

ical violaceous papules on the skin. Oral erythema multiforme is often accompanied by skin erythema or target lesions. Herpes simplex virus infection tends to occur on the vermilion border of the lower lip and usually manifests in a younger person.

HOW TO MAKE THE DIAGNOSIS

Punch biopsy of the skin or oral lesions demonstrates the intraepidermal blister. An additional biopsy for immunofluorescence microscopy of adjacent normal skin or mucosa (sent in Michel's transport media to a special laboratory) demonstrates intraepidermal deposition of immunoglobulin, usually IgG. Indirect immunofluorescence of the serum measures circulating antibodies to basement membrane. The titer often correlates with the disease activity. However, a positive indirect immunofluorescence study alone is not sufficient for diagnosis.

TREATMENT

Systemic corticosteroids, such as prednisone, 1 to 2 mg/kg daily, is usually required for PV. Patients with PF may respond to lower doses of oral corticosteroids. Corticosteroid-sparing regimens for either PV or PF include oral niacinamide, 500 mg three times daily, plus tetracycline, 500 mg three times daily, or intramuscular gold, 50 mg weekly. Other approaches include immunosuppressive and cytotoxic agents such as azathioprine, mycophenolate, methotrexate, or cyclophosphamide. Treatment is continued for months to years.

PROGNOSIS

Untreated PV can be fatal when complicated by infection or fluid imbalance. PF has a better prognosis, and patients rarely die from it. In both PV and PF, it is possible for spontaneous resolution to occur in some patients after 3 to 5 years.

CHAPTER 31

Toxic Epidermal Necrolysis/Stevens–Johnson Syndrome (ICD-9 695.1)

Jeffrey P. Callen, M.D.

SYMPTOMS AND SIGNS

Toxic epidermal necrolysis (TEN) and Stevens–Johnson syndrome (SJS) are two terms that describe the clinical spectrum of a severe, life-threatening, blistering disorder of the skin and mucous membranes. Historically, more extensive skin loss (greater than 30% of body surface) is labeled TEN, whereas SJS is usually associated with less than 10% of body surface skin loss (see Chapter 16). In TEN/SJS, there is often a 1- to 3-day prodrome period of fever, conjunctivitis, pharyngitis, or pruritus. Frank skin pain and tenderness constitute an ominous sign. Mucosal surfaces of the mouth, eyes, genitalia, and anus are affected early in the disease (Fig. 31-1). Shortly thereafter, the patient develops widespread bullae that are easily ruptured; target lesions may also be seen (Fig. 31-2). The bullae can be extended laterally when pressed down upon, or the skin may tear when it is rubbed (Nikolsky's sign). TEN/SJS may progress dramatically to sheets of skin loss (Fig. 31-3).

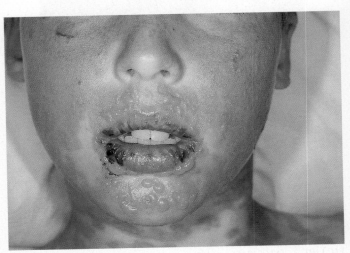

FIGURE 1. TEN/SJS. Mucosal blisters and erythematous patches on the skin.

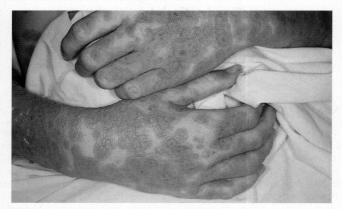

FIGURE 2. TEN/SJS. Target lesions and bullae on the hands and arms of the patient in Figure 31-1.

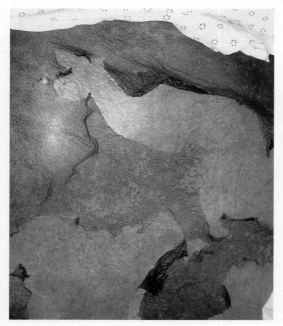

FIGURE 3. TEN/SJS. Skin is lost in sheets in severe cases.

Fluid and electrolyte balance, poor thermoregulation, and bacterial infections may result from the skin loss. Skin healing occurs with dyspigmentation but minimal, if any, scarring. Ocular involvement can result in blindness.

TEN and SJS are rare disorders and almost always are a manifestation of an adverse drug reaction. The most common offending drugs are antibiotics (sulfonamides, penicillins, cephalosporins), anticonvulsants (phenytoin, phenobarbital, carbamazepine), nonsteroidal antiinflammatory agents, and allopurinol. Many other drugs have been implicated, including systemic corticosteroids. TEN/SJS occurs more commonly in HIV-infected individuals or in those on any immunosuppressive or cytotoxic therapy.

DIFFERENTIAL DIAGNOSIS

TEN and SJS are distinctive and dramatic once they are manifest fully. Early in their evolution, they may be confused with erythema multiforme, paraneoplastic pemphigus, or a morbilliform drug eruption. Other blistering diseases must also be considered, particularly if there is an atypical presentation. Staphylococcal scalded skin syndrome, which occurs most often in children, is more superficial and can be distinguished on skin biopsy.

HOW TO MAKE THE DIAGNOSIS

Punch biopsy can help confirm the clinical diagnosis of TEN/SJS.

TREATMENT

TEN and SJS are usually drug-related, and suspect drugs should be stopped. Patients must often be attended in a burn center with careful attention to infection and fluid and electrolyte balance. Many approaches to dressing and cleansing have been championed in the literature. However, none has been tested in a scientific manner or adequately compared. Ophthalmologic examination and early intervention may prevent scarring and blindness.

Drug treatment is controversial. Corticosteroids, to be useful, must be given in high doses; methylprednisone, 2 mg/kg per day intravenously the first 24 to 72 hours, may help. Cytotoxic or immunosuppressive therapies are unproven. Plasmapheresis has also been suggested as part of early management. Intravenous immunoglobulin, 0.75 g/kg per day for 4 to 5 days, has recently been demonstrated to result in rapid control and speedy healing.

PROGNOSIS

Mortality is 30% overall, but higher in elderly patients with multiple preexisting medical conditions.

CHAPTER 32

Seborrheic Keratosis (ICD-9 702.19)

James C. Shaw, M.D.

SYMPTOMS AND SIGNS

Seborrheic keratoses are most often asymptomatic and only occasionally pruritic. They can manifest as solitary or multiple lesions. Common sites include the head, neck, and back. They are usually verrucous, scaling, and sharply differentiated from surrounding skin (Fig. 32-1). The color can vary from flesh-colored to black or even red, if irritated or inflamed. Seborrheic keratoses can be flat or raised and range in size from less than 0.5 cm to more than 3 cm in diameter. Slow enlargement over years is normal. Rarely, rapid development of multiple lesions occurs (Leser-Trélat sign) and can be a paraneoplastic phenomenon associated with gastric and other adenocarcinomas. A variant, called **dermatosis papulosa nigra,** appears as multiple small, dark seborrheic keratoses on the face of African Americans. Stucco keratoses are multiple, white 0.2- to 0.4-cm seborrheic keratoses on the lower legs or arms.

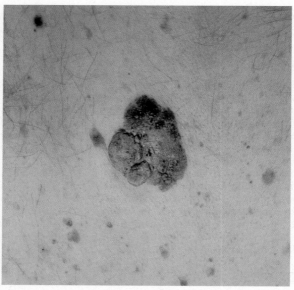

FIGURE 1. Seborrheic keratosis. Verrucous, scaling, light brown, "stuck-on" lesion.

DIFFERENTIAL DIAGNOSIS

Common warts have a more papillomatous surface with many black dots visible on their surface. These are thrombosed vessels. Squamous cell carcinoma-in-situ (Bowen's disease) is a reddish-brown patch of hyperkeratosis, often on sun-exposed skin. Rarely, a black seborrheic keratosis can resemble malignant melanoma.

HOW TO MAKE THE DIAGNOSIS

Diagnosis of seborrheic keratosis is clinical. Excisional biopsy is necessary if malignant melanoma is suspected.

TREATMENT

Treatment for seborrheic keratosis is generally not required and tends to be for cosmetic purposes. Methods include cryotherapy, electrodesiccation, and curettage, or shave excision.

PROGNOSIS

Untreated lesions persist and may enlarge slowly over years. Large lesions can become traumatized, pruritic, or rarely secondarily infected. There appears to be no risk of malignant degeneration beyond that of normal skin.

CHAPTER 33

Squamous Cell Carcinoma (ICD-9 173.3

head, ear; 173.4 scalp, neck; 173.5 trunk; 173.6 upper

extremity; 173.7 lower extremity)

David H. Frankel, M.D.

SYMPTOMS AND SIGNS

Squamous cell carcinoma of the skin (SCC) is often asymptomatic, although patients may complain of itching or pain. SCC appears as a scaling, hyperkeratotic papule or nodule (Fig. 33-1). It is usually on sun-exposed skin and may ulcerate. Occasionally, SCC develops in sites of chronic inflammation or ulceration, as in discoid lupus erythematosus or hidradenitis suppurativa, or in sites of radiation therapy or burn. In these instances, the clinical appearance may be more subtle. Such SCC are at high risk for recurrence or metastasis. Other high-risk sites are the lower lip, ear, digits, scalp, and penis. Recurrent SCC must also be considered in the high-risk group.

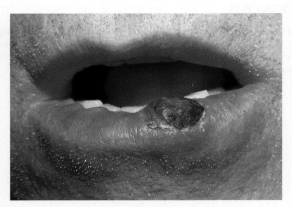

FIGURE 1. Squamous cell carcinoma. High-risk lesion on the lip.

DIFFERENTIAL DIAGNOSIS

Keratoacanthoma may be undistinguishable from SCC, unless it has the characteristic central keratin plug. Seborrheic keratoses appear greasy, "stuck on," and warty. Verrucae are also scaling but, when shaved, reveal the tell-tale black dots of thrombosed vessels.

HOW TO MAKE THE DIAGNOSIS

Punch biopsy or shave biopsy is needed to confirm the diagnosis of SCC.

TREATMENT

Data on cure rates of various therapies for SCC are difficult to summarize because the number of variables and risk factors is great. Cure rates for all modalities are nearly 90% when the modality suits the type of SCC being treated. Cryotherapy or electrodesiccation and curettage should be used only for superficial, small, low-risk lesions. Surgical excision and primary closure, the time-honored method, is more likely to be curative for higher-risk lesions and has the advantage that excision margins can be evaluated by the pathologist. Remember that excised lesions with positive margins must be reexcised until margins are negative. Mohs' micrographic surgery is reserved for high-risk lesions, in which the cure rate—even for difficult tumors—can be as high as 95%. Radiation therapy is generally reserved for large lesions in the elderly.

PROGNOSIS

The risk of local recurrence after treatment is greatest for SCC in high-risk sites or in SCCs that are large (over 1 cm in diameter), poorly differentiated, or invasive to the deep dermis or fat, or that have invaded the perineurium. Overall, the 5-year rate of metastasis is approximately 5% for SCC on sun-damaged skin. Rates are higher for high-risk tumors. About one third of patients with SCC develop another SCC within 5 years. Affected patients should have yearly follow-up to check for recurrence, new tumors, or lymph node metastasis.

CHAPTER 34
Actinic Keratosis (ICD-9 702.2)
David H. Frankel, M.D.

SYMPTOMS AND SIGNS

Actinic keratoses (AK), in general, are asymptomatic. Sometimes patients complain of itching or burning. These symptoms should be considered signs of possible transformation to squamous cell carcinoma (SCC). AK present as small, 3- to 6-mm, red, rough, poorly circumscribed patches on sun-exposed skin (Fig. 34-1). Common sites include the nose, tips of the ears, forehead, forearms, and hands. AK are extremely common in the elderly, although given the population growth in the US sunbelt, it is not uncommon to see them in young adults. Most AK do not progress to SCC and, with scrupulous sun protection, some resolve spontaneously. Lesions that grow rapidly, ulcerate, thicken, or become symptomatic should be held in suspicion as possible early SCCs.

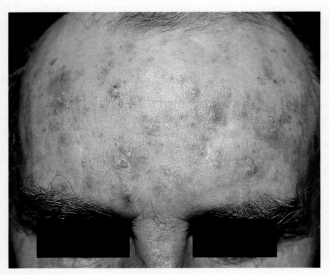

FIGURE 1. Actinic keratoses. Multiple, red, scaling, poorly circumscribed lesions on sun-exposed skin.

The equivalent of AK on the lip, actinic cheilitis, is a premalignant condition characterized by loss of the vermilion border, milky discoloration, and scaling—most often on the lower lip.

DIFFERENTIAL DIAGNOSIS

Occasionally, small patches of eczema or psoriasis may look like AK. In general, however, eczema is more pruritic than AK and psoriasis is unlikely to be limited to sun-exposed areas, especially because sunlight ameliorates psoriasis.

HOW TO MAKE THE DIAGNOSIS

Finding typical lesions on sun-exposed skin is enough to make the diagnosis of AK. Punch or shave biopsy is recommended when SCC is suspected.

TREATMENT

AK that do no resolve within 1 month should be treated with light cryotherapy or light electrodesiccation and curettage. Fluorouracil solution 2% or 5%, or cream 5%, applied twice daily for up to 3 weeks may be used for patients with numerous lesions. Patients should be warned that fluorouracil often causes contact dermatitis and photosensitivity. Actinic cheilitis can be treated similarly to AK, but carbon dioxide laser vermilionectomy is often the most effective method for treating the entire lower lip.

PROGNOSIS

Patients with AK respond well to therapy. However, they are likely to develop new lesions, and yearly follow-up is reasonable.

CHAPTER 35
Keratoacanthoma (ICD-9 238.2)
James C. Shaw

SYMPTOMS AND SIGNS

Keratoacanthomas (KA) are usually asymptomatic and develop rapidly over 2 to 6 weeks. The rapid enlargement of a dome-shaped nodule of up to 1 cm in diameter with a central keratin-filled plug is typical (Fig. 35-1). KA usually appear on sun-exposed areas of the face, neck, arms, and hands. Rare syndromes exist in which multiple keratoacanthomas develop. The Ferguson–Smith type of KA consists of multiple, large KA; the Gryzbowski type consists of multiple, eruptive small lesions.

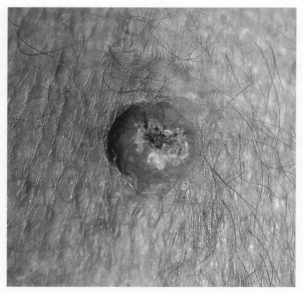

FIGURE 1. Keratoacanthoma. Rapidly developing, dome-shaped papule or nodule with central keratin plug on sun-damaged skin.

DIFFERENTIAL DIAGNOSIS

Squamous cell carcinoma (SCC) can appear identical to keratoacanthoma, but the growth of SCC is usually slower. Molluscum contagiosum can resemble small keratoacanthomas, but molluscum lesions usually remain small—2 to 3 mm in diameter.

HOW TO MAKE THE DIAGNOSIS

Diagnosis of KA is usually made by history and examination. However, if SCC is a possibility, a shave or excisional biopsy must be done to confirm the diagnosis.

TREATMENT

KA may resolve spontaneously, leaving depressed, atrophic scars. However, because of the clinical and histologic similarity to SCC, plus rare reports of metastases, most authors consider KA to be a variant of SCC and therefore treat KA with ablative therapies. The treatment of choice is excision. Alternatives include intralesional methotrexate, 5-fluorouracil, or interferon α-2a, systemic retinoids (especially for multiple keratoacanthomas), or radiation therapy.

PROGNOSIS

Complete excision is usually curative. Recurrences can develop at the site of treated lesions.

CHAPTER 36

Basal Cell Carcinoma (ICD-9 173.3 head, ear;
173.4 scalp, neck; 173.5 trunk; 173.6 upper extremity; 173.7
lower extremity)
James C. Shaw. M.D.

SYMPTOMS AND SIGNS

The presentation of basal cell carcinoma (BCC), the most common human cancer, is an asymptomatic papule that often goes unnoticed by patients. The typical presentation is an enlarging papule or a sore that does not heal and bleeds easily—the so-called "rodent ulcer" (Fig. 36-1). The sun-exposed areas of the head and neck are the most common sites involved. A papule or plaque with a pearly or translucent appearance and crossed by telangiectasias is highly suggestive. Superficial BCCs resemble a patch of dermatitis with a pearly rim (Fig. 36-2). Sclerosing BCCs are insidious and hard to diagnose. They are white to yellow and often indistinguishable from common scar tissue (Fig. 36-3). Pigmented BCCs resemble nodular malignant melanoma (Fig. 36-4). Patients who received therapeutic radiation for acne or tinea capitis are at high risk for the development of multiple BCCs.

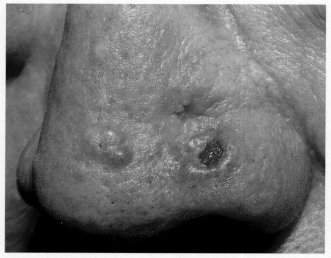

FIGURE 1. Basal cell carcinoma. "Rodent ulcer" (left nostril) next to typical pearly papule with telangiectasias.

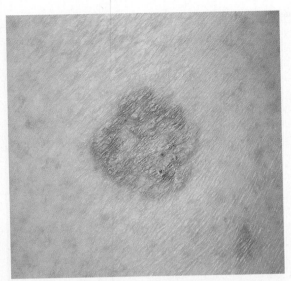

FIGURE 2. Superficial basal cell carcinoma resembles dermatitis, but with raised, pearly border.

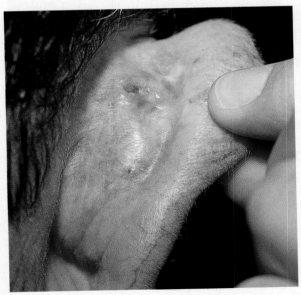

FIGURE 3. Sclerosing basal cell carcinoma can be mistaken for scar tissue.

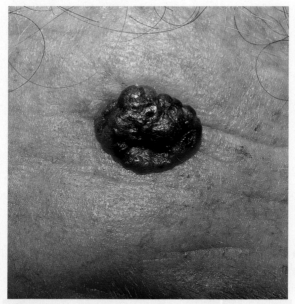

FIGURE 4. Pigmented basal cell carcinoma resembles nodular malignant melanoma.

DIFFERENTIAL DIAGNOSIS

Flesh-colored nevi can resemble BCCs, as can other benign lesions such as neurofibromas, hidrocystomas, and lichen planus–like keratoses. Hyperkeratotic BCCs can be confused with squamous cell carcinoma.

HOW TO MAKE THE DIAGNOSIS

Most BCCs can be suspected by physical examination with magnification and good lighting. Histologic confirmation by either shave or punch biopsy is indicated to confirm the diagnosis and assess histologic subtypes, which include nodular, sclerosing, and superficial types.

TREATMENT

Treatment options for BCC include surgical excision, Mohs' micrographic surgery, radiation therapy, and destructive modalities such as electrodesiccation and curettage or cryotherapy. Although there is literature to support all modalities, the best method is probably surgical excision, because this allows histologic confirmation of excision margins. Remember that excised lesions with positive margins must be re-excised. Mohs' micrographic surgery is indicated for high-risk lesions about the central face and ears, for sclerosing BCCs, for recurrent BCCs, and for BCCs with aggressive histologic features. Radiation therapy is reserved for elderly patients.

PROGNOSIS

The combined cure rate of primary BCCs is greater than 90% and greater than 95% with Mohs' surgery. For recurrent BCCs, Mohs' surgery has a 5-year cure rate of approximately 94%, compared with 90% for radiation, 83% for excision, and 60% for electrodesiccation and curettage. It is worthwhile to remember that nearly one third of patients with BCCs develop another BCC within 5 years. This is especially common in patients with a history of radiation therapy. BCCs rarely metastasize.

CHAPTER 37

Melanocytic Nevus (ICD-9 216.3 face; 216.4 scalp; 216.5 trunk; 216.6 upper extremity; 216.7 lower extremity)

David H. Frankel, M.D.

SYMPTOMS AND SIGNS

Junctional, compound, and intradermal nevi are benign lesions and should not be symptomatic. Symptoms such as itching or pain may indicate transformation to malignant melanoma (MM). **Junctional nevi** are usually macules, although sometimes they are slightly elevated. **Compound nevi** are macules or papules. **Intradermal nevi** are papular. Both lesions are symmetric, have sharp borders, and are uniformly pigmented tan to dark brown or even black (Fig. 37-1). Intradermal nevi may be nonpigmented, pink, or tan (Fig. 37-2). They too are sharp-bordered, measure 1 to 6 mm in diameter, and do not undergo rapid enlargement or other sudden changes in appearance.

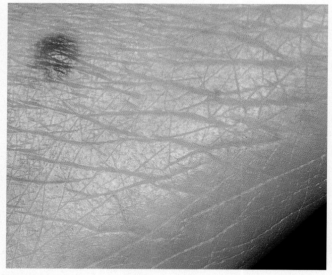

FIGURE 1. Melanocytic nevus. This compound nevus on the foot is symmetric, sharply bordered, uniformly pigmented, 3 mm in diameter, and without a history of rapid enlargement.

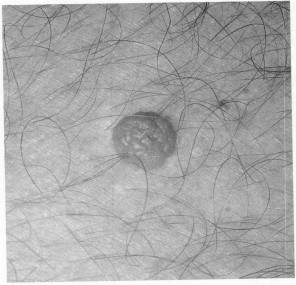

FIGURE 2. Melanocytic nevus. Intradermal nevus with no ABCDE changes.

DIFFERENTIAL DIAGNOSIS

There are many benign pigmented lesions to consider in the differential diagnosis of melanocytic nevi, including dermatofibroma, lentigo, angioma, postinflammatory hyperpigmentation, skin tag, and others. Any lesions with "ABCDE" features must be biopsied to rule out MM (**ABCDE: A**symmetry, **B**order irregularity, **C**olor variegation, **D**iameter greater than 6 mm, **E**nlargement over a 1- or 2-month period; see Chapter 39 on MM). Most benign nevi appear before age 35 years. Pigmented lesions appearing in persons older than 35 should be suspected of being MM.

HOW TO MAKE THE DIAGNOSIS

If the lesion is asymptomatic and there are no ABCDE changes, the diagnosis can be made clinically. If MM is suspected, the diagnosis must be made by excisional biopsy.

TREATMENT

Benign nevi are removed for cosmetic reasons. This can be accomplished by shave, punch, or elliptical technique.

PROGNOSIS

Melanocytic nevi are benign lesions that may become MMs at any time. Patients should be taught the importance of self-examination and early signs of MM.

CHAPTER 38

Halo Nevus (ICD-9 M8723/0)

John T. Crissey, M.D.

SIGNS AND SYMPTOMS

Itching and varying degrees of erythema may precede or accompany the development of the characteristic depigmented ring of the halo nevus (HN). The halo is several millimeters to centimeters wide and surrounds a preexisting pigmented nevus (Fig. 38-1). The halo usually reaches its maximum size in 1 or 2 months, after which the central nevus slowly diminishes in size and over a period of months or years tends to disappear. The depigmented area eventually resumes its normal color. The condition is common and usually occurs in children and young adults. The incidence of HN is high—nearly 25%—in patients

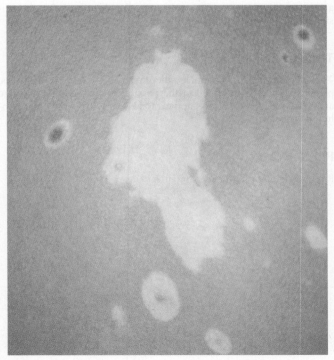

FIGURE 1. Halo nevus surrounded by zones of depigmentation; patient also has a large patch of vitiligo.

with vitiligo, and HN may be a forerunner of that disease. HN is a benign junctional, dermal, or compound nevocellular nevus undergoing morphologic and pathologic changes in response to an immunologic process not yet fully understood.

DIFFERENTIAL DIAGNOSIS

Zones of depigmentation can occur around malignant melanoma, blue nevus, dermatofibroma, and neurofibroma.

HOW TO MAKE THE DIAGNOSIS

When the clinical picture of HN is typical, the history and appearance should suffice. If the central nevus shows signs suggestive of malignant melanoma—asymmetry, irregular border, variations in color, diameter greater than 6 mm, or a history of sudden growth—an excisional biopsy is indicated.

TREATMENT

Typical cases need no treatment other than reassurance. Nevertheless, patients should be informed of the possibility of developing vitiligo and reexamined at 6-month intervals for 1 year to be certain that resolution is occurring.

PROGNOSIS

Repigmentation usually takes months to years.

CHAPTER 39

Malignant Melanoma (ICD-9 172.3 head, ear; 172.4 scalp, neck; 172.5 trunk; 172.6 upper extremity; 172.7 lower extremity)

James C. Shaw, M.D.

SYMPTOMS AND SIGNS

Malignant melanoma (MM) is usually asymptomatic. Sometimes it can cause pruritus. Pruritus in a "mole" is a cardinal symptom that cannot be ignored. Bleeding is also an important complaint. MM usually develops as a patch, papule, or nodule. It is almost always pigmented, although nonpigmented (**amelanotic MM**) forms can arise. MM develops in preexisting nevi or de novo on normal skin. It is estimated that by the year 2000, nearly one in 75 Americans will develop MM during their lifetime. The **ABCDE** of diagnosis are crucial to both physicians and patients (Figs. 39-1 through 39-3):

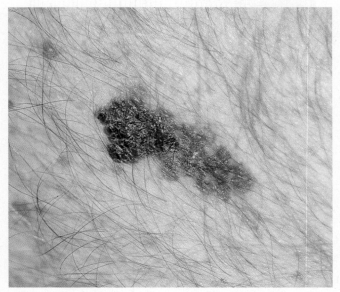

FIGURE 1. Malignant melanoma. **A**symmetry, **B**order irregularity, **C**olor variegation, **D**iameter, **E**nlargement (by history) of malignant melanoma.

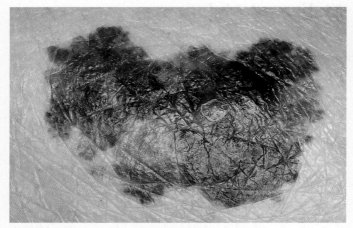

FIGURE 2. ABCD all present in this malignant melanoma.

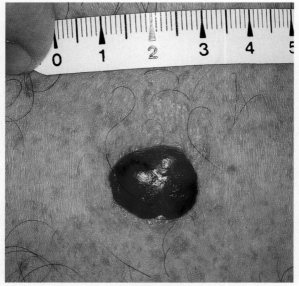

FIGURE 3. Rapidly growing nodular malignant melanoma.

Asymmetry
Border irregularities
Color variegation, including blue, gray, red, and black
Diameter usually greater than 6 mm
Enlargement, either of an existing nevus or of a new lesion, over a 1- or 2-month period

DIFFERENTIAL DIAGNOSIS

Darkly pigmented seborrheic keratoses, pigmented basal cell carcinomas, and darkly pigmented atypical nevi commonly resemble MM. Pyogenic granulomas resemble amelanotic melanoma. Blue nevi, common in Asians, also look like MM.

HOW TO MAKE THE DIAGNOSIS

Histologic confirmation is essential for the diagnosis of MM. Biopsies must include epidermis, dermis, and subcutaneous fat. Excisional biopsy is preferable, but incisional biopsy is indicated in large lesions, especially when MM is suspected in large facial lesions. Shallow shave biopsies should not be done. A shave may not reach to the base of the lesion; therefore, the precise millimeter of depth of tumor invasion cannot be estimated. Knowledge of depth of invasion is essential for proper staging and treatment (see Prognosis). Sentinel lymph node biopsy is increasingly used in patients with a proven melanoma greater than 1 mm deep. This method uses dye and isotope mapping to disclose the sentinel node.

TREATMENT

Surgical excision of primary cutaneous melanoma is the treatment of choice for MM. Current recommendations on margins are 0.5 cm for melanoma in situ (epidermal only), 1 cm for MM less than 1.5 mm deep, 1 to 2 cm for lesions 1.51 to 4 mm deep, and 2 to 3 cm for lesions deeper than 4 mm. Lymph node dissection is indicated when there is proven metastasis to a single drainage basin, and in some cases of intermediate depth (1.5 mm to 4 mm deep). Chemotherapy and immunologic therapies are used as adjuvant and palliative measures.

Preventive measures are vital. Sun protection beginning in infancy may be the most effective measure. Sun-protective behavior includes avoidance of direct sun exposure, especially between 10 AM and 3 PM, and careful use of protective clothing, hats, and sun blocks. Skin self-examination for early detection is also important, especially for patients with numerous moles or with the atypical mole syndrome.

Monthly total body examination with lighting and mirrors or with assistants often detect early lesions that can be cured.

PROGNOSIS

Depth of tumor invasion is the best predictor of long-term survival. Approximate 5-year survival figures are over 95% for tumors 0.75 mm deep, 85% for tumors 0.76 to 1.49 mm, 75% for tumors 1.50 to 2.49 mm, 65% for tumors 2.5 to 3.99, and 45% for tumors deeper than 4 mm. Five-year survival drops to 35% if there is nodal involvement and 5% if there is distant metastasis. Younger patients and women may have more favorable outcomes. MM on the hands, feet, or mucosa have a worse prognosis.

CHAPTER 40

Dysplastic Nevus (ICD-9 238.9)

James C. Shaw. M.D.

SYMPTOMS AND SIGNS

Dysplastic nevi (DN), also called atypical nevi, are asymptomatic. Patients may have only a single lesion or hundreds of them. DN are macules at least 5 mm in diameter with variable pigmentation, indistinct margins, and irregular, asymmetric outline (Fig. 40-1). Pigmentation frequently includes shades of brown and red and occasionally some black. The pigment variability is usually less than what is seen with malignant melanoma. The most common site is the back. Patients with many lesions (**dysplastic nevus syndrome**) have DN anywhere on the trunk and also on the proximal extremities and scalp (Fig. 40-2). Pruritus or bleeding may be associated with transformation to melanoma.

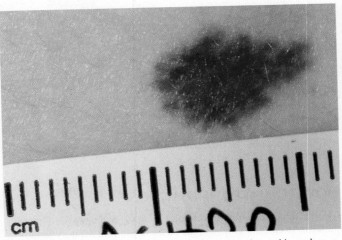

FIGURE 1. Dysplastic nevus with variegated pigmentation and irregular borders. Malignant melanoma was ruled out by excisional biopsy.

DIFFERENTIAL DIAGNOSIS

Common melanocytic nevi are sometimes irregularly pigmented, but more typically tan to dark brown. They also have distinct margins, regular outlines, and raised contour and measure less than 5 mm in diameter. **Halo nevi** are surrounded by a white ring of depigmentation. Malignant melanomas have many of the features of dysplastic nevi, and

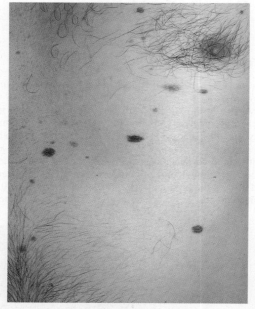

FIGURE 2. Patient with the dysplastic nevus syndrome presenting with many lesions on the trunk.

may be impossible to differentiate from dysplastic nevi on clinical examination.

HOW TO MAKE THE DIAGNOSIS

Clinical features often are enough to make a diagnosis. However, punch or excisional biopsy of the entire lesion is mandatory for any lesion that appears suspicious for malignant melanoma. Destructive treatments such as cryotherapy, electrodesiccation, and carbon dioxide laser ablation are contraindicated because they will not provide histologic confirmation of the diagnosis.

TREATMENT

Patients should be taught the "ABCDE" of malignant melanoma, the importance of sun protection, and the need to examine themselves every month. They should also be examined by their physician every 6 to

12 months. The use of selected or total body photography has been recommended in patients with large numbers of lesions.

Reexcision of DN with positive margins is controversial when there is significant malanocyte atypia. However, because the histologic diagnosis of DN is often made in the presence of only minimal atypia, close communication with the consulting dermatopathologist is essential to make sure DN are neither overtreated nor undertreated.

PROGNOSIS

Patients with multiple dysplastic nevi have an increased risk of developing melanoma. With a family history of melanoma as well, the relative risk is even greater. These patients must be carefully watched.

CHAPTER 41

Dermatofibroma (ICD-9 216.9)

James C. Shaw, M.D.

SYMPTOMS AND SIGNS

Patients present with an asymptomatic smooth, firm, round, brownish papule or nodule, usually measuring less than 1 cm in diameter (Fig. 41-1). There is often a peripheral rim of hyperpigmentation. When dermatofibromas (DF) are pinched, they dimple in the center. DF are most common on the legs of women. They are thought to be fibrosing reactions to a local insult such as an arthropod bite or folliculitis.

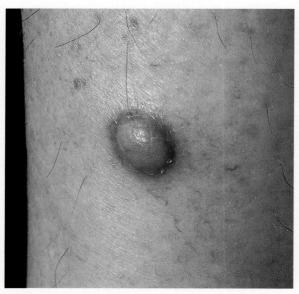

FIGURE 1. Dermatofibroma. Firm, brown papule with peripheral rim of hyperpigmentation.

DIFFERENTIAL DIAGNOSIS

Scars or keloids, if small and round, can mimic DF. They do not dimple, however. Melanocytic nevi, melanomas, and solitary lesions of Kaposi's sarcoma can resemble a darkly pigmented dermatofibroma. In larger lesions, usually greater than 2 cm, dermatofibrosarcoma protuberans (DFSP) needs to be considered. DFSP is a locally aggressive malignant fibrosing neoplasm.

HOW TO MAKE THE DIAGNOSIS

Most DF are detected by examination alone. The "dimple" is very helpful. A history of an unchanging lesion present for months to years supports the diagnosis. Punch or elliptical biopsy extending to subcutaneous fat is indicated if the diagnosis is in doubt.

TREATMENT

No treatment is necessary. In patients in whom the lesion causes symptoms such as pain or bleeding with leg shaving or if for cosmetic reasons it is unacceptable, the treatment is surgical excision and primary closure.

PROGNOSIS

DF persist if not removed.

CHAPTER 42
Skin Tags (ICD-9 701.9)
Charles A. Gropper, M.D.

SYMPTOMS AND SIGNS

Skin tags are asymptomatic. They are extremely common, small (1 to 3 mm) flesh-colored or brown papules. They are usually pedunculated (Fig. 42-1). Skin tags can occur anywhere on the body, but are partic-

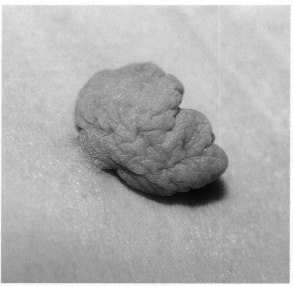

FIGURE 1. Skin tag. Soft, flesh-colored, pedunculated papule.

ularly common around the neck, in the groin or axillae, or under the breasts of women. They occur more often in people who are obese and tend to run in families.

DIFFERENTIAL DIAGNOSIS

Skin tags can be confused with seborrheic keratoses, neurofibromas, or nevi. Seborrheic keratoses often have a bumpy surface. Neurofibromas tend to be compressible and larger than skin tags. Nevi frequently are larger than skin tags and more darkly pigmented.

HOW TO MAKE THE DIAGNOSIS

The diagnosis is made on examination. It can be confirmed by shave biopsy.

TREATMENT

Skin tags that are asymptomatic are treated mainly for cosmetic reasons. Additional reasons for treating skin tags include color change, bleeding, itching, and interference with clothing. The lesions may be removed by shearing at the base with a scalpel or scissors. They can also be destroyed by light electrodesiccation or cryosurgery.

PROGNOSIS

Skin tags are benign lesions. Like any other skin growth or area of skin, they can rarely be the site of development of a malignancy so change of color should not be ignored. Any person who has a few skin tags will likely develop more as time progresses.

CHAPTER 43
Epidermoid Cyst and Pilar Cyst
(ICD-9 706.2)

Charles A. Gropper

SYMPTOMS AND SIGNS

Cysts are asymptomatic until they become inflamed. They are among the most common skin lesions. Patients present with subcutaneous nodules that have the consistency of semifirm jelly, much like the feel of an eyeball. They are freely movable under the skin. Epidermoid cysts appear most commonly on the face, neck, upper trunk, and scrotum. They often have a visible central punctum (Fig. 43-1). Pilar cysts occur mainly on the scalp; multiple cysts are common. Pilar cysts often lack a central punctum. Cysts are filled with keratin, which may have a slightly cheesy smell. Either type can rupture

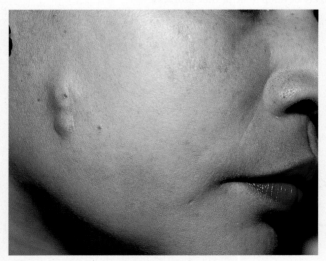

FIGURE 1. Epidermoid cysts on face. Note central punctum on upper lesion.

and become inflamed; frank infection with *Staphylococcus aureus* is less common. In either situation, the lesions become quite painful and drain serous or foul-smelling keratinaceous material.

DIFFERENTIAL DIAGNOSIS

Furuncles can be easily confused with inflamed epidermoid cysts. Carcinomas of the lung, breast, and genitourinary system can metastasize to the scalp. These lesions, however, are firm and fixed.

HOW TO MAKE THE DIAGNOSIS

The diagnosis is suggested by the appearance and consistency of the lesion. The presence of a punctum is especially helpful. Diagnosis can be confirmed only by removal.

TREATMENT

Asymptomatic cysts need not be removed if they do not trouble the patient. It is helpful to remove cysts that become inflamed, but removal should be undertaken only after the inflammation has subsided for several weeks. Inflamed cysts often respond to high-dose oral erythromycin, 500 mg two to four times daily because of its antiinflammatory properties, and warm compresses. Alternatively, the lesions can be incised and drained or injected with a small amount (less than 0.5 mL) of intralesional triamcinolone acetonide solution in a concentration of 2.5 to 5.0 mg/mL. Infected cysts are treated the same as furuncles.

PROGNOSIS

The prognosis of epidermoid cysts is variable. Some spontaneously regress, some persist without change, and some continue to grow. The particular course of any given lesion is not predictable. Although epidermoid cysts are always benign, there are extremely rare reports of cysts giving rise to squamous cell carcinoma.

CHAPTER 44

Molluscum Contagiosum (ICD-9 078.0)

John T. Crissey, M.D.

SYMPTOMS AND SIGNS

Molluscum contagiosum (MC) is an asymptomatic condition. Lesions are skin-colored, white, or slightly pink, flattened globose papules, 3 to 6 mm in diameter, many with a small central aperture or dell (Fig. 44-1). The surface is "semigloss," pearl-like, and waxy. Lesions may occur singly or in groups. Exposed surfaces are favored, but no area is exempt. Groin and genitalia are commonly involved in sexually active persons. Lesions undergoing spontaneous resolution often become acutely inflamed. Facial involvement in adults usually indicates concomitant HIV infection. Lesions in these cases may become very large and run together. MC is a viral infection, is common in children and young adults, and is spread by skin to skin contact.

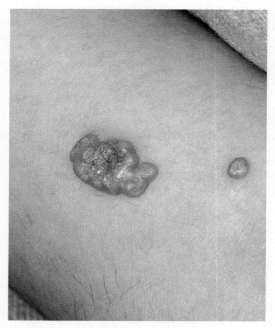

FIGURE 1. Molluscum contagiosum. Giant molluscum in a patient with AIDS. Note smaller, more typical lesion with central dell.

DIFFERENTIAL DIAGNOSIS

MC can be mimicked in immunocompromised patients by skin lesions of disseminated cryptococcosis, histoplasmosis, and other deep mycoses.

HOW TO MAKE A DIAGNOSIS

The distinctive appearance of MC usually suffices. Direct examination of the whitish, curd-like content of the lesions mounted in 15% KOH solution, or smeared on a slide and Giemsa-stained, shows the large intracytoplasmic inclusions characteristic of the disease ("molluscum bodies"). Atypical presentations in immunocompromised patients need punch or shave biopsy confirmation.

TREATMENT

Lesions few in number can be curetted easily. Anesthesia is seldom necessary. Cryotherapy with liquid nitrogen is effective. More aggressive treatment is indicated in immunocompromised patients. Laser ablation as well as electrodesiccation and curettage are the procedures of choice.

PROGNOSIS

For children, the prognosis is excellent. Resolution of MC even without treatment usually occurs in 3 to 9 months. For HIV-infected persons, the prognosis is guarded. Many cases are resistant even to aggressive treatment.

CHAPTER 45

Cherry Angioma (ICD-9 228.01)

Lawrence Charles Parish, M.D.

SYMPTOMS AND SIGNS

Cherry angiomas are asymptomatic lesions. Patients often become worried about the appearance of small (1 to 10 mm) red papules (Fig. 45-1). The lesions are benign and appear during early middle age, most commonly on the trunk.

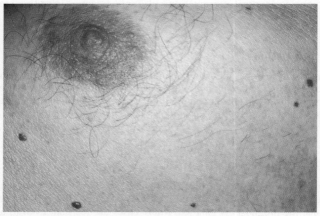

FIGURE 1. Cherry angiomas. Small, red papules on the trunk that blanch with pressure.

A key clinical feature is that the red color disappears with direct pressure applied under a glass microscope slide or by pulling taut the surrounding skin.

DIFFERENTIAL DIAGNOSIS

Cherry angiomas are sometimes confused with insect bites or irritated seborrheic keratoses.

HOW TO MAKE THE DIAGNOSIS

The diagnosis of cherry angioma is clinical.

TREATMENT

The lesions are easily removed by snipping with an iris scisssors followed by light electrodesiccation of the base.

PROGNOSIS

Cherry angiomas do not disappear on their own. Generally, a few form every year or so.

C H A P T E R 4 6

Granuloma Annulare (ICD-9 695.89)

Lawrence Charles Parish, M.D.

SYMPTOMS AND SIGNS

Granuloma annulare (GA) is an asymptomatic condition. It begins as flat-topped to pinpoint firm red papules, 1 to 3 mm in diameter, which gradually enlarge to create a coin-like appearance (Fig. 46-1). The lesions are usually on the dorsal aspects of the hands and feet but may be found on the face, buttocks, ankles, wrists, and elbows. Sometimes GA persists for several years and can involve most of the body—disseminated granuloma annulare. Other forms of GA are rare: a plaque type that is flat and infiltrated, resembling necrobiosis lipoidica; an erythematous type that has red papules as the predominant morphology; a subcutaneous type that presents as subcutaneous nodules; and the perforans type, which ulcerates.

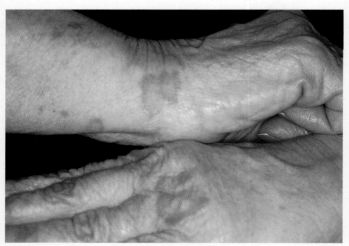

FIGURE 1. Granuloma annulare. Red papules that gradually enlarge to coin-like lesions.

DIFFERENTIAL DIAGNOSIS

Annular GA may be confused with the annular form of sarcoidosis in which the lesions are predominantly facial, especially the nose. Tinea infections are scaling. Nodular GA on the elbows may be confused with rheumatoid nodules. Plaque GA resembles necrobiosis lipoidica.

HOW TO MAKE THE DIAGNOSIS

The diagnosis of GA is made by the characteristic clinical appearance. Confirmation may be obtained by punch biopsy. Biopsy is the only way to diagnose the subcutaneous variety.

TREATMENT

Most therapy is minimally effective. Super-potent topical corticosteroid ointments or creams can be used. The old adage that a biopsy makes the lesion disappear is stretching the truth.

PROGNOSIS

GA usually disappears within a few years but it can last several years. It should not leave any scars.

CHAPTER 47

Folliculitis (ICD-9 704.8)

Lawrence Charles Parish, M.D.

SYMPTOMS AND SIGNS

Folliculitis is asymptomatic or causes mild itching or tenderness. Although the follicular red papules and pustules can be found anywhere there are hair follicles, the lesions are most often seen on the beard, neck, chest, buttocks, and thighs (Fig. 47-1). Occasionally, the inflammation is severe enough to create crusting and pain. The condition is an infection of the hair follicles. *Staphylococcus aureus* is the most common culprit. *Pseudomonas aeruginosa* is responsible for hot tub dermatitis. In this condition, the follicular lesions are predominantly on the trunk and buttocks.

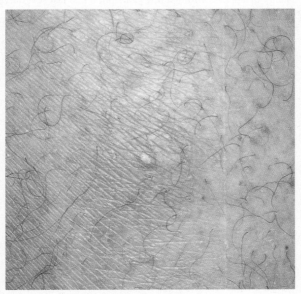

FIGURE 1. Folliculitis. Mildly pruritic, erythematous follicular pustule.

DIFFERENTIAL DIAGNOSIS

Pustules from *Candida albicans* are distinguished by fungal cultures. Viral exanthems are usually accompanied by fever and other systemic manifestations.

HOW TO MAKE THE DIAGNOSIS

Folliculitis is a clinical diagnosis. Sometimes, it can be confirmed by a bacteriologic culture, although the pathogen is frequently not recovered.

TREATMENT

Because the inflammatory process is often minimal and the infection is superficial, topical antimicrobials such as mupirocin ointment 2% may be applied twice daily. Extensive skin disease or involvement of hairy areas requires oral antibiotic therapy such as dicloxacillin, 250 mg three to four times daily, or erythromycin, 250 mg three to four times daily. If resistance develops, ciprofloxacin, 500 mg twice daily may be needed. Occasionally, washing with an antibacterial solution such as chlorhexidine 4% or applying a benzyl peroxide 5% gel twice daily will stop the process. A low-potent topical corticosteroid cream twice daily is also helpful.

PROGNOSIS

Folliculitis may usually be prevented by frequent washing with soap and avoiding occlusive lotions and pomades.

CHAPTER 48

Pyogenic Granuloma (ICD-9 686.1)

Lawrence Charles Parish, M.D.

SYMPTOMS AND SIGNS

Pyogenic granuloma (PG) ranges from asymptomatic to tender and painful. It may also bleed. Common sites are fingers, toes, lips, buccal mucosa, anal mucosa, and the upper aspects of the trunk. PGs measure 5 to 10 mm in diameter, are red to black (depending on trauma), and are often pedunculated, irritated, and friable (Fig. 48-1). PGs develop

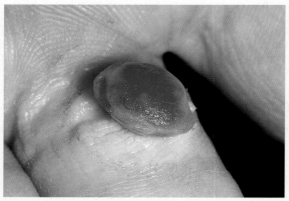

FIGURE 1. Pyogenic granuloma. Red, friable, pedunculated papule, which developed during pregnancy.

within a few weeks of injury to the site; they may also be caused by pregnancy or systemic retinoids. Despite the name, they are neither bacterial infection nor granulomatous, but are simply benign vascular hyperplasias. PG are more common in children and young adults. They almost never involute spontaneously.

DIFFERENTIAL DIAGNOSIS

The clinical picture of PG is characteristic. However, an irritated nevus or seborrheic keratosis might be confused with a PG. Malignant melanoma may have the same appearance if it is pedunculated. Occasionally, an embedded tick may look like a PG.

HOW TO MAKE THE DIAGNOSIS

The history of easy bleeding and the clinical appearance of PG are usually sufficient for the diagnosis.

TREATMENT

A PG is easily removed by shaving the lesions and lightly electrodesiccating the base.

PROGNOSIS

Once a PG is removed, there should be no recurrence. The lesion itself does not cause scarring.

CHAPTER 49

Milium (ICD-9 706.2)

John T. Crissey, M.D.

SYMPTOMS AND SIGNS

Milium is a tiny asymptomatic keratinous cyst, the cause of which is unknown. Its clinical appearance is a round or oval, white or yellowish body directly beneath the surface of the skin. Milia are common. They occur singly or in groups and measure only 1 to 2 mm in diameter (Fig. 49-1). Cheeks, eyelids, forehead, temples, penis, scrotum, and the internal aspect of the labia minora are the favored sites. All age groups are affected. Facial milia can be found in 50% of newborn infants; these lesions disappear spontaneously in a few weeks. Similar lesions in older children and adults sometimes disappear without treatment, but usually persist indefinitely.

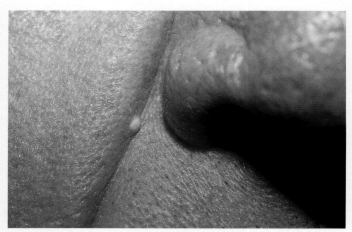

FIGURE 1. Milium. Tiny, thin-walled papule filled with yellow keratin.

Milia may appear de novo or in association with the healing of the lesions of other cutaneous problems, particularly vesiculobullous disorders—pemphigus vulgaris, epidermolysis bullosa, second-degree burns, porphyria cutanea tarda, bullous pemphigoid, and bullous lichen planus. Milia may also follow abrasions, radiation therapy, and dermabrasion.

DIFFERENTIAL DIAGNOSIS

The closed comedones of acne vulgaris sometimes resemble milia.

HOW TO MAKE THE DIAGNOSIS

The clinical appearance of milia is distinctive. Expression of the contents, a small whitish semisoft ball of keratinous debris, confirms the diagnosis.

TREATMENT

Contents of milia are easily removed by opening the lesions with a cutting edge needle or a pointed scalpel blade and expressing the contents with a comedo extractor or by squeezing gently with the thumb and forefinger.

PROGNOSIS

Once removed, milia usually do not recur.

CHAPTER 50

Syringoma (ICD-9 M8407/0)

David H. Frankel, M.D.

SYMPTOMS AND SIGNS

Syringomas are asymptomatic. Patients are often concerned about their cosmetic effect. They occur predominantly in women and begin during puberty. Most syringomas appear on the eyelids as 1 to 3 mm in diameter, soft, white to yellowish translucent papules (Fig. 50-1). They usually occur in crops and may also appear on the cheeks and trunk.

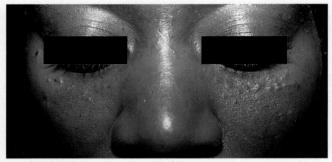

FIGURE 1. Syringoma. Tiny, translucent, white to yellow papules on lower eyelids with crops of lesions under left eye.

DIFFERENTIAL DIAGNOSIS

Papules of acne vulgaris are erythematous and usually not limited to the lower eyelid.

HOW TO MAKE THE DIAGNOSIS

The diagnosis of syringoma is made by examination.

TREATMENT

Treatment of syringoma is for cosmetic purposes only. Various destructive methods such as light electrodesiccation and carbon dioxide laser ablation may be effective.

CHAPTER 51

Furuncle (ICD-9 680.7) and Carbuncle
(ICD-9 680.9)

John T. Crissey, M.D.

SYMPTOMS AND SIGNS

Furuncles are painful and exquisitely tender. The cliché, "sore as a boil," is accurate. The furuncle is a *Staphylococcus aureus* infection seated deeply in a pilosebaceous unit. When two or more adjacent units are involved, the lesion is called a carbuncle. A firm erythematous nodule about 1 cm in diameter enlarges for several days, becomes fluctuant, points, and ruptures to drain a mixture of necrotic tissue and creamy pus streaked with blood (Fig. 51-1). Healing usually takes place in 1 or 2 weeks. A depressed saucer-like scar may result. Any area of the skin bearing hair follicles may be attacked, but the favored sites are areas subject to friction and sweating—buttocks, axillae, groin, face, and neck. In the carbuncle, initial redness and nodularity is more extensive. The lesion is larger, 6 to 8 cm in diameter. Pointing and drainage occur at several sites simultaneously. The carbuncle has a special predilection for the nape of the neck. Carbuncles heal much more slowly than furuncles.

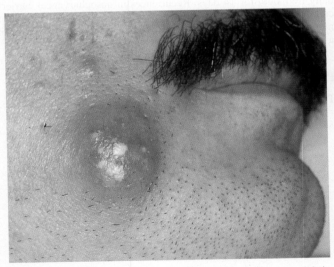

FIGURE 1. Furuncle. Exquisitely tender, fluctuant, erythematous nodule in infected hair follicle.

DIFFERENTIAL DIAGNOSIS

Inflamed and ruptured epidermoid and pilar cysts sometimes resemble furuncles. History of a preexisting nodule and the characteristic pasty, rancid-smelling contents of these lesions serve to differentiate them from the furuncle or carbuncle. Early lesions of hidradenitis suppurativa may resemble furuncles.

HOW TO MAKE A DIAGNOSIS

The clinical picture of furuncle and carbuncle is distinctive. Identification of the *Staphylococcus* in Gram-stained smears or cultures of the pus establishes the diagnosis in atypical presentations.

TREATMENT

Incision and drainage of individual furuncles may suffice. Systemic antibiotics shorten the course and are mandatory in immunocompromised patients and in all patients with carbunculosis. Dicloxacillin and cephalexin are the medications of choice. A suitable dicloxacillin dosage schedule is 250 to 500 mg four times daily by mouth for 10 to 14 days. Cephalexin can be given in doses of 250 to 500 mg four times daily by mouth for 14 days. Recurrences in nasopharyngeal carriers can be minimized by the twice-daily intranasal application of mupirocin or bacitracin ointments. Resistant and recurrent cases merit a search for immune dysfunction.

PROGNOSIS

The prognosis is excellent in the absence of immunologic compromise.

CHAPTER 52

Erythema Nodosum (ICD-9 695.2)

John T. Crissey, M.D.

SYMPTOMS AND SIGNS

Erythema nodosum (EN) is usually painful and tender. It is a reactive, inflammatory panniculitis that appears as indurated, erythematous, nodules that can be single or multiple. The lesions are 1 to 20 cm in diameter and hot to the touch. Older lesions often have a bluish, brownish, yellow-green, or purplish tinge and resemble contusions (Fig. 52-1). Borders are not sharply demarcated. Extensor surfaces of the lower leg, thigh, and ankle are the favored sites, although arms and other areas are occasionally affected. When multiple, EN nodules are usually bilateral, but not necessarily symmetric. Fever, arthralgia, and malaise may accompany or precede the eruption. The disease is much more common in women than men.

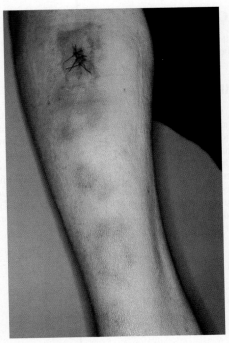

FIGURE 1. Erythema nodosum. Painful nodules on the shins resemble contusions. (Biopsy site at top)

Most cases of EN occur in association with streptococcal infections or sarcoidosis. Behçet's syndrome, coccidioidomycosis, Crohn's disease, histoplasmosis, leprosy, lymphogranuloma venereum, lymphomata, psittacosis, pulmonary tuberculosis, and ulcerative colitis are also known causes, as well as medications, especially sulfonamides, iodides, and oral contraceptives. In many cases, the cause remains obscure.

The course of EN is variable. Lesions usually involute in a few weeks, but EN associated with chronic disease may persist or recur for many months.

DIFFERENTIAL DIAGNOSIS

Cellulitis is usually not nodular, although pain and warmth are common. Insect bites, urticaria, lupus panniculitis, and erythema multiforme may be nodular and easily confused with EN.

HOW TO MAKE THE DIAGNOSIS

The clinical picture of EN is distinctive. Punch biopsy, deep enough to include subcutaneous fat, is indicated in atypical cases.

TREATMENT

Treatment should be directed against the cause, which must be searched for assiduously in every case. Bed rest, elastic bandages, and aspirin or nonsteroidal antiinflammatory agents to tolerance are helpful. Injection of 0.1 to 0.5 mL of triamcinolone acetonide suspension, 5 mg/mL, directly into the nodules is a practical and effective approach when lesions are few in number. EN usually responds rapidly to systemic corticosteroids, but these agents are often contraindicated in the diseases that cause the eruption. Potassium iodide (SSKI) by mouth, five to six drops three times daily for 2 to 3 weeks, is sometimes remarkably effective.

PROGNOSIS

Prognosis is good when the underlying disease can be controlled. Recurrences are common in idiopathic EN.

CHAPTER 53

Hidradenitis Suppurativa (ICD-9 705.83)

John T. Crissey, M.D.

SYMPTOMS AND SIGNS

In hidradenitis suppurativa (HS), painful, tender, erythematous, nodular lesions appear in the axillary, genital, and perianal areas (Fig. 53-1). Open comedones and patulous follicular orifices in and about the inflammatory areas are hallmarks of the disease. HS usually begins at a single site, but eventually appears in other apocrine gland-bearing areas as well. In severe cases, buttocks, thighs, periumbilical areas, nipples, and scalp may be involved. Nodules suppurate, point, rupture, and drain pus, blood, and serous exudates. Sinus tracts form. Scarring is prominent. The disease progresses in fits and starts. HS is due to recurrent bacterial infection of apocrine glands (apocrine acne) and is primarily a disease of young adults. HS is sometimes associated with cystic acne vulgaris, occasionally with pilonidal sinuses or with Crohn's disease.

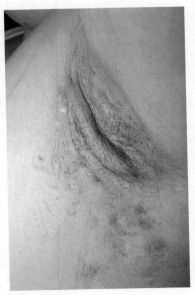

FIGURE 1. Hidradenitis suppurativa. Painful, tender nodules in apocrine areas such as the axilla.

DIFFERENTIAL DIAGNOSIS

Initial acutely inflamed lesions of HS are indistinguishable from furunculosis. The short course and complete resolution of the latter serve to differentiate the two conditions. The deep mycoses, scrofuloderma, lymphogranuloma venereum, and granuloma inguinale (donavanosis) may all mimic HS.

HOW TO MAKE THE DIAGNOSIS

The diagnosis of HS is made clinically. The long history of recurrences and presence of scarring is especially helpful.

TREATMENT

The choice of systemic antibiotics for treating HS is guided by results of culture and sensitivity. *Staphylococcus aureus* is the organism primarily responsible for HS. However, multiple antibiotics may be necessary when *S. aureus,* streptococci, *Escherichia coli, Proteus,* or *Pseudomonas* strains are also isolated. Intralesional injections with triamcinolone acetonide are definitely helpful. A dose of 0.1 to 0.3 mL of a 5 to 10 mg/mL suspension can be injected into nonfluctuant sites every 2 or 3 weeks for several months. Incision and drainage of fluctuant nodules are indicated. Excision of fibrotic nodules and sinus tracts is often successful. Intractable disease involving large areas may require complete excision and skin grafting.

PROGNOSIS

Prognosis is good for control, less promising for cure. HS tends to diminish and may even involute completely as the patient approaches middle age.

CHAPTER 54

Chondrodermatitis Nodularis Chronica Helicis (ICD-9 380.0)

John T. Crissey, M.D.

SIGNS AND SYMPTOMS

Tenderness is the hallmark of chondrodermatitis nodularis chronica helicis (CNCH). Patients pull away when the lesion is touched, and they are often awakened at night when they roll over and the pillow comes into contact with the area. Some lesions are subject to sudden episodes of intense pain not associated with contact of any kind. CNCH is a chronic disease of the skin of the ear, which presents as one or several small, dome-shaped, skin-colored or erythematous papular excrescences, usually at the apex of the helix or anthelix (Fig. 54-1). An adherent scale overlying a central horny plug is evident in the typical lesion. The right ear is more often involved than the left. CNCH is largely a disease of the middle-aged and elderly. Males are more commonly affected than females. The cause is thought to be localized trauma from excessive telephone use, earphones, head bands, and the like, although clear-cut evidence for such is seldom present.

DIFFERENTIAL DIAGNOSIS

Molluscum contagiosum lesions, verruca vulgaris, actinic keratoses, and the tophi of gout may resemble CNCH. None of these approach CNCH in lesional tenderness.

HOW TO MAKE THE DIAGNOSIS

The history, location, appearance, and tenderness of the lesions combine to render this an easy diagnosis. Histopathology is characteristic. When doubt exists, a punch or shave biopsy can be diagnostic.

TREATMENT

Removal of sources of trauma is indicated when they are known. Excision, desiccation and curettage, and ablation with carbon dioxide and argon lasers, all have been used with success. Intralesional injections with an insoluble corticosteroid such as triamcinolone acetonide are sometimes effective; 0.1 to 0.3 mL of a 5 to 10 mg/mL suspension can be injected into the base of the lesion once monthly for 2 or 3 months.

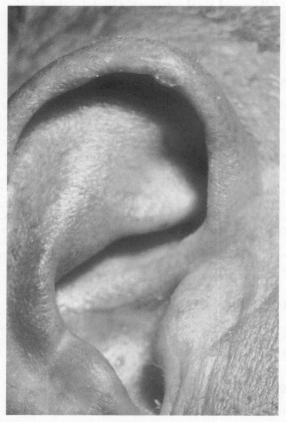

FIGURE 1. Chondrodermatitis nodularis chronica helicis. Painful papule on the helix of the ear.

PROGNOSIS

Prognosis is good, but recurrences are common after all forms of treatment.

CHAPTER 55

Keloid (ICD-9 701.4) and Hypertrophic Scar (ICD-9 701.4)

John T. Crissey, M.D.

SYMPTOMS AND SIGNS

Both hypertrophic scars and keloids have a tendency to itch; keloids are sometimes tender and painful. They are overgrowths of fibrous tissue at the sites of trauma or inflammatory disease processes. Keloids and hypertrophic scars present as firm papular or nodular lesions. Shoulders, upper trunk, ear lobes, chin, neck, and the lower part of the legs are the favored sites.

Keloids begin in a site of trauma, but continue to grow for prolonged periods of time, often extending many centimeters beyond the initial site to form large elevated mesa-like plaques (Fig. 55-1). Keloids may also appear as knobby individual lesions, dome-shaped nodules that resemble cobblestones, or irregular shiny plaques from which ridge-like

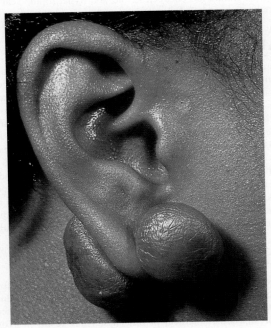

FIGURE 1. Keloid extending far beyond point of ear piercing.

bands and cords extend like pseudopods. The surface may be reddish or purplish at first and later hyper- or hypopigmented. Lesions located over joints can seriously interfere with function. Keloid susceptibility is sometimes familial; the condition is more common in dark-skinned individuals.

Hypertrophic scars tend to follow the shape of original trauma, such as linear incisions, suture tracks, and circumscribed burn areas. They usually reach a certain size and stop growing.

DIFFERENTIAL DIAGNOSIS

Fibromata, pigmented basal cell carcinomata, and the skin lesions of sarcoidosis sometimes resemble keloids.

HOW TO MAKE THE DIAGNOSIS

Location and morphology point to the proper diagnosis. A punch biopsy confirms the clinical diagnosis if doubt exists. In many instances, differentiation between keloid and hypertrophic scar can be made only after extended observation.

TREATMENT

No completely satisfactory treatment is available. Intralesional injections with an insoluble corticosteroid, such as triamcinolone acetonide suspension, are helpful in softening lesions and relieving pain and tenderness. A dose of 0.1 to 0.3 mL of a 20 mg/mL suspension can be injected into several lesional sites once monthly for 3 or 4 months. Cryotherapy with liquid nitrogen is useful for smaller lesions. Results with laser ablation are encouraging. Surgical excision of ear lobe keloids is often successful, but excision of lesions in other areas is usually followed by prompt recurrence unless combined with adjuvant treatments such as radiation, compression, or intralesional corticosteroids. As a preventive measure, the prolonged application of silicone sheets postoperatively to surgical wounds in patients with a tendency to develop keloids or hypertrophic scars has been helpful.

PROGNOSIS

Prognosis is good for improvement with treatment, but poor for a totally satisfactory result. Some keloids and hypertrophic scars diminish in size with the person's age. Patients should be aware that unnecessary procedures, whether medical or otherwise, may result in avoidable lesions.

CHAPTER 56

Lipoma (ICD-9 214.9)

John T. Crissey, M.D.

SYMPTOMS AND SIGNS

Lipomas are asymptomatic in most cases, although larger lesions that impinge on nerves are sometimes painful. A lipoma presents as a palpable, ill-defined, sometimes lobulated, soft or doughy mass, a "miniature pillow beneath the skin" (Fig. 56-1). Lipomas are mobile and not fixed to the overlying skin. They are common and usually make their initial appearance in early middle age. Size varies. Most are small, 2 or 3 cm in diameter, although lesions of long duration can be many centimeters in diameter.

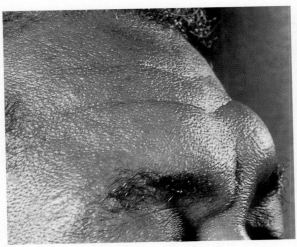

FIGURE 1. Lipoma. Soft, doughy mass under the skin.

Growth is slow. Neck, shoulders, and back are the most common sites involved, but no area is exempt. Skin overlying the lesion is normal in appearance, occasionally slightly pigmented. Lipomas are usually solitary or few in number, although they occur in large numbers in familial multiple lipomatosis, an autosomal dominant condition. This condition usually begins in early adulthood.

DIFFERENTIAL DIAGNOSIS

Deep-seated epidermal inclusion cysts sometimes mimic lipomas.

HOW TO MAKE A DIAGNOSIS

Location, mobility, and consistency point to the proper diagnosis. Needle aspiration biopsy confirms the diagnosis in doubtful cases.

TREATMENT

Total excision is curative, although not necessary for these benign lesions. Large lipomas associated with deeper anatomic structures may be difficult to excise. Liposuction has been successful in the eradication of smaller lesions.

PROGNOSIS

Lipomas are benign and remain so. Most stabilize at some point and stop enlarging.

CHAPTER 57

Xanthelasma (ICD-9 272.2)

John T. Crissey, M.D.

SYMPTOMS AND SIGNS

Asymptomatic flat or slightly raised, yellow to yellow-orange plaques appear on the eyelids, particularly on the nasal side (Fig. 57-1). Small at first, the lesions slowly enlarge, and in some cases progress to involve virtually the entire lid. Most patients with xanthelasma are middle-aged or older. Xanthelasma in patients younger than 30 years is usually a sign of significant disturbances in lipoprotein metabolism. In about 60% of patients, xanthelasma is a normolipoproteinemic xanthoma with no demonstrable systemic cause. Nevertheless, these lesions may be associated with hyperlipoproteinemias that can result in atherosclerotic cardiovascular disease.

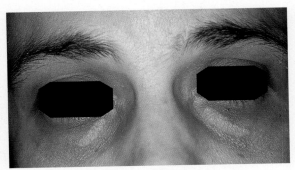

FIGURE 1. Xanthelasma. Yellow plaques on lower eyelids.

DIFFERENTIAL DIAGNOSIS

Eyelid milia of unusual size can resemble the lesions of xanthelasma.

HOW TO MAKE A DIAGNOSIS

Location and distinctive color combine to confirm the diagnosis of xanthelasma. All patients with xanthelasma should be checked for hyperlipoproteinemia.

TREATMENT

The lesions can be treated successfully with electrodesiccation, excision, carbon dioxide laser ablation, or careful application of 35% trichloroacetic acid solution.

PROGNOSIS

The prognosis is excellent in normolipoproteinemic cases, guarded when associated with hyperlipoproteinemia.

CHAPTER 5 8

Xanthoma (ICD-9 272.2)

John T. Crissey, M.D.

SYMPTOMS AND SIGNS

Xanthomata are asymptomatic lesions. The most important of these lesions commonly encountered in practice are those associated with genetically based disturbances in lipoprotein metabolism, namely, the familial forms of hypercholesterolemia, dyslipoproteinemia, combined hyperlipoproteinemia, and hypertriglyceridemia. Xanthelasma (see Chapter 57) and arcus senilis, a gray ring at the periphery of the cornea, are sometimes seen in these disorders. Palpable and visible lesions appear in several distinctive forms.

Eruptive xanthomata appear suddenly as crops of small, asymptomatic, discrete, dome-shaped papules on the buttocks and thighs. Arms, elbows, knees, and palms may also be involved. Reddish at first, the lesions soon take on a yellowish or yellowish-brown color (Fig. 58-1). Some are surrounded by a reddish halo. Papules may run together to form plaques. **Eruptive xanthomata** may occur in hyperlipoproteinemias secondary to other metabolic diseases, especially poorly controlled diabetes mellitus.

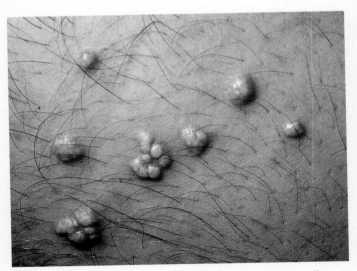

FIGURE 1. Eruptive xanthoma appear as red papules that become yellow or yellow-brown with time.

Xanthoma tendinosum presents as firm, nontender, subcutaneous nodules associated with tendons. The Achilles and patellar tendons, and extensor tendons of the hands are the favored sites. Overlying skin is usually normal in appearance, occasionally yellowish.

Xanthoma tuberosum presents as smooth, nontender, yellowish papules and nodules on the elbows and knees.

Xanthoma striatum palmare lesions are yellow to yellow-orange infiltrations along the palmar and digital flexural creases, often accompanied by papular xanthomata on the palms.

DIFFERENTIAL DIAGNOSIS

Keloids resemble old, tuberous lesions in darker-skinned patients but are preceded by trauma. Cutaneous sarcoid is usually more waxy in appearance, but may be indistinguishable.

HOW TO MAKE THE DIAGNOSIS

The yellow color and characteristic morphology usually permit the diagnosis of xanthoma to be made at sight. Punch biopsy findings are distinctive and confirm the clinical diagnosis when doubt exists.

TREATMENT

Management depends on the exact nature of the causative metabolic disturbance. A complete lipid workup is essential. Therapy includes dietary restrictions, weight control, and pharmacologic measures to control lipid levels.

PROGNOSIS

Xanthomata usually respond satisfactorily to treatment. Early recognition and control of the underlying metabolic disturbances can also significantly reduce the incidence and severity of cardiovascular problems with which the genetic lipoprotein disturbances are closely linked.

CHAPTER 59
Warts (ICD-9 078.1)
John T. Crissey, M.D.

SYMPTOMS AND SIGNS

Warts are generally asymptomatic. They are caused by human papilloma virus (HPV) infections of skin and mucocutaneous surfaces. All lesions are potential sources of infection. They appear in several different forms.

Verruca Vulgaris

Verruca vulgaris is the common wart that usually occurs on the hands, fingers, wrists, and forearms of children and young adults. Nail folds are often involved. No area is immune to infection. The lesions are asymptomatic, flat or dome-shaped papules, 2 to 10 mm in diameter (Fig. 59-1). They may run together to form still larger lesions. Early verrucae are usually smooth. Mature lesions are rough; the surface becomes covered with tiny keratotic projections. Warts may be skin-colored, yellowish, brown, or dark gray. They sometimes occur in linear configurations, the virus having been inoculated in a scratch "like planting a row of potatoes" (Koebner's phenomenon).

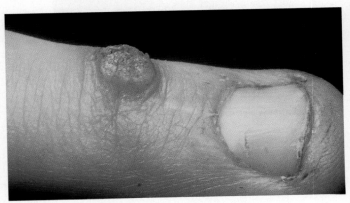

FIGURE 1. Verruca vulgaris on the finger.

Verruca Plantaris (Plantar Warts)

Unlike other verrucae, plantar lesions are often tender and sometimes painful. They usually appear at the pressure points on the sole, where callus formation often obscures the true nature of the lesion. Trimming the callus reveals a whitish sodden circle studded with dark red or black dots (thrombotic capillaries), a sign that is virtually diagnostic. Larger lesions may also show evidence of pressure-induced intralesional hemorrhage. Multiple plantar verrucae may run together to produce mosaic-like patterns, sometimes involving almost the entire sole.

Verruca Plana (Flat Warts)

Verruca plana are usually seen on the face or dorsum of the hands in young people. They are skin-colored, pinkish or brownish, sharply marginated, flat papules, 1 to 3 mm in diameter (Fig. 59-2). Surface of

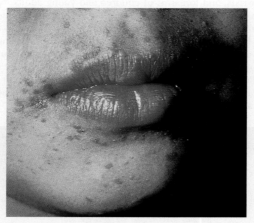

FIGURE 2. Verruca plana. Smooth, brown, flattened papules are often on the face.

the papules is relatively smooth. The lesions are discrete, scattered irregularly or distributed in groups. Linear configurations (Koebner's phenomenon) are common.

Verruca Filiformis

Filiform verrucae are single or multiple, small, slender, thread-like projections with a frayed keratotic tip. They usually occur on the eyelids, nares, and other parts of the face, occasionally on the neck.

Condyloma Acuminatum

Condylomata acuminata present as exuberant, pink to red, moist, papular warts on mucocutaneous surfaces, particularly the genitalia, perianal area, and crural folds (Fig. 59-3). They bleed easily and are often foul-smelling. Lesions on adjacent skin surfaces may assume the clinical form of verruca vulgaris. Condylomata are usually contracted through sexual contact. They spread rapidly in pregnancy. Several of the strains of the HPV that cause condylomata predispose patients to cervical dysplasia, cervical, vulvar, anal, or penile squamous cell carcinoma. In children, condylomata are sometimes a sign of sexual abuse.

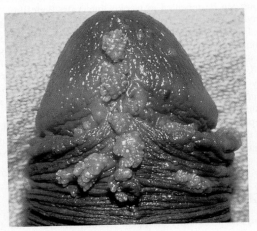

FIGURE 3. Condyloma acuminata on the penis.

DIFFERENTIAL DIAGNOSIS

Skin tags can mimic verruca filiformis. Large callouses can be mistaken for verruca plantaris. Condyloma latum lesions of secondary syphilis sometimes resemble condyloma acuminatum.

HOW TO MAKE A DIAGNOSIS

Most forms of verrucae are diagnosable at sight from the morphology alone. Trim the callus over plantar lesions and look for the characteristic black dots. Histopathology is distinctive; punch or excision biopsy can confirm the clinical diagnosis in atypical presentations.

TREATMENT

No true antiviral therapy is available. All active treatment is an assault designed to ablate the virus and its captive host tissue completely or stimulate a favorable immune response. Assault techniques commonly used include liquid nitrogen cryotherapy, light electrodesiccation, curettage, laser ablation, and application of salicylic acid plasters.

When few in number, condylomata acuminata are best treated with electrodesiccation. For more extensive cases, topical applications of podophyllin, podofilox, or imiquimod are useful. A 15% to 25% solution of podophyllin in compound tincture of benzoin is applied to the condylomata and washed off in 2 hours. To avoid excessive reaction treatment should be confined to a 5 to 6 cm^2 area at each sitting. Applications can be repeated at weekly intervals. Podofilox, gel 5%, a podophyllin relative marketed in kits, can be applied at home by the patient. Podofilox is applied with a cotton-tipped swab every 12 hours for 3 consecutive days and then withheld for 4 days. These cycles can be repeated four times. Podofilox is contraindicated in pregnancy. Imiquimod, marketed as a 5% cream, is applied sparingly to the condylomata by the patient three times per week at bedtime and washed off with soap and water 6 to 10 hours later. It is continued until a satisfactory result is obtained, but for no more than 16 weeks.

Prompt gynecologic consultation is indicated when condylomata appear on the genitalia during pregnancy. Infants delivered vaginally in this situation can develop recurrent respiratory papillomatosis in later life.

PROGNOSIS

Most verrucae eventually disappear whether treated or not. Condylomata acuminata are less likely to do so.

CHAPTER 60

Kaposi's Sarcoma (ICD-9 176.0)

Jeffrey P. Callen, M.D.

SYMPTOMS AND SIGNS

No specific symptoms are associated with Kaposi's sarcoma (KS). KS occurs in two forms—one related to aging (classic form) and another due to immune suppression (acquired or iatrogenic). The classic form most often occurs on the legs and consists of violaceous patches, papules, or plaques (Fig. 60-1). This form is more prevalent in persons of Mediterranean and Jewish ancestry. KS associated with immuno-suppression occurs in any site and is often mistaken for a simple ecchymosis. KS is a vascular neoplasm associated with human herpesvirus-8 infection.

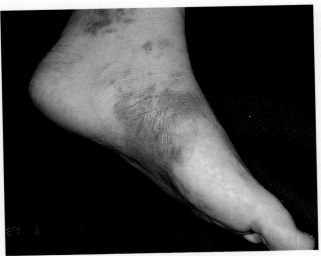

FIGURE 1. Classic Kaposi's sarcoma presenting as nonblanching violaceous patches and papules on the lower extremities.

DIFFERENTIAL DIAGNOSIS

Ecchymoses are not papular or indurated. Neither are telangiectasias. Bacillary angiomatosis must be a considered in differential diagnosis, particularly in the HIV-infected individual.

HOW TO MAKE A DIAGNOSIS

Punch biopsy confirms the diagnosis. Systemic KS should be excluded by a chest roentgenogram and computed tomography of the abdomen.

THERAPY

In the elderly patient with classic KS, therapy with local irradiation is often effective. Vinblastine or other antineoplastic agents are used for systemic disease. For immunosuppressed patients, therapy should aim to improve immune function. Patients with HIV-associated KS often respond to combinations of newer antiretroviral therapies. For organ transplantation patients, the condition often remits as immunosuppressive therapy is eased.

PROGNOSIS

Patients with classic KS and localized disease have an excellent prognosis. In immunosuppressed patients or patients with disseminated disease, death due to this neoplasm is possible from bleeding, infection, or dysfunction of vital organs.

CHAPTER 61

Ecchymosis (ICD-9 459.89)/Actinic Purpura (ICD-9 287.2)

Jeffrey P. Callen, M.D.

SYMPTOMS AND SIGNS

Ecchymoses are asymptomatic or tender nonpalpable hemorrhages, usually 1 cm or more in diameter. They usually follow trauma, even mild trauma. The lesions are often linear or angulated and tend to occur on the dorsal hands, extensor forearms, pretibial area, and anterolateral thighs. The most common form of ecchymotic hemorrhage, actinic purpura, occurs on the sun-damaged skin of the elderly (Fig. 61-1).

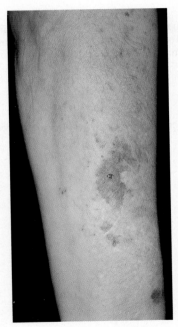

FIGURE 1. Actinic purpura on sun-damaged skin of the forearm.

DIFFERENTIAL DIAGNOSIS

Considerations include deficiencies of vitamin C or vitamin K, disseminated intravascular coagulopathy, leukemia, immune thrombocytopenia purpura, hemophilia, Kaposi's sarcoma, Ehlers–Danlos syndrome, von Willebrand's disease, and anticoagulant, corticosteroid systemic or topical), and aspirin therapy. Domestic violence must also be considered.

HOW TO MAKE THE DIAGNOSIS

Clinical examination is usually sufficient for diagnosis of ecchymosis/actinic purpura. Biopsy is rarely necessary. The history should assess the use of drugs and dietary habits. Laboratory testing, if necessary, should include platelet count, prothrombin time, partial thromboplastin time, and bleeding time.

THERAPY

No treatment is needed for actinic purpura. Vitamin K–containing creams are of unproven benefit. Prevention of trauma may help prevent further lesions. Treatment of any underlying conditions may reverse the process.

PROGNOSIS

Ecchymoses are benign, and usually resolve within weeks.

CHAPTER 62

Cutaneous Vasculitis (ICD-9 446.20)

Jeffrey P. Callen, M.D.

SYMPTOMS AND SIGNS

Patients with vasculitis may complain of burning or pain in the affected areas. The condition is often accompanied by systemic involvement, manifested as arthralgias, myalgias, fever, abdominal pain, or hematochezia. Palpable purpura is the most common cutaneous sign (Fig. 62-1). However, urticarial lesions, ulcerations, nodules, or livedo reticularis (a bluish discoloration in a net pattern) can also occur. Palpable purpura or urticarial lesions are more common in small blood vessel disease, whereas medium-sized vessel involvement manifests as livedo reticularis, nodules, or ulcers. Vasculitis may be a sign of many underlying conditions, including infections (bacterial endocarditis, acute respiratory infections, hepatitis B or C), drug reactions (from aspirin, penicillin, sulfonamides, or others), cryoglobulinemia, collagen vascular disorders (systemic lupus erythematosus, rheumatoid arthritis, or Sjögren's syndrome), lymphoproliferative disorders and Henoch–Schönlein purpura.

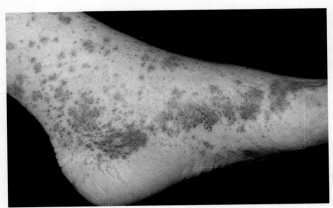

FIGURE 1. Cutaneous vasculitis with palpable purpura due to ampicillin.

DIFFERENTIAL DIAGNOSIS

Patients with purpuric lesions from cholesterol emboli often have a history of recent angiography. Capillaritis or thrombocytopenia cause purpura that is nonpalpable. Urticarial vasculitis is an unusual condition that should be suspected when individual lesions persist beyond 24 hours. Insect bite reactions and physical urticarias must also be considered.

HOW TO MAKE THE DIAGNOSIS

The diagnosis of cutaneous vasculitis is confirmed by punch biopsy. The best site for biopsy is a fresh lesion, preferably less than 24 hours old. When assessing the possibility of medium-sized vessel involvement, a deeper and larger biopsy is often required. In patients with an obvious cause, testing is directed toward determining systemic involvement: renal function tests, urinalysis, and chest x-ray. In patients without an identifiable cause, laboratory assessment should include blood cultures (in patients with fever), paraproteins, cryoproteins, hepatitis C viral antibody, antinuclear antibody, and serologies for lupus erythematosus and rheumatoid factor.

TREATMENT

Therapy for cutaneous vasculitis ranges from observation with symptomatic therapy to aggressive immunosuppressive agents. Drug-associated vasculitis usually resolves when the offending agent is stopped. Patients with chronic cutaneous vasculitis may respond to oral colchicine, 0.6 mg twice daily; dapsone, 100 to 200 mg daily; low-dose methotrexate, 10 to 25 mg weekly; or azathioprine, 1 to 2 mg/kg daily. Systemic corticosteroids may be useful, but steroid-related toxicity is common and whenever possible these agents should be avoided. Patients with hepatitis C–associated vasculitis may be treated effectively with antiviral regimens including interferon α2a 3 million units subcutaneously three times per week and ribavirin 1,000 to 1,200 mg per day orally for 24 to 48 months. Henoch–Schönlein purpura is treated symptomatically.

PROGNOSIS

The prognosis of cutaneous vasculitis is dependent on the degree of systemic involvement and the severity of underlying diseases.

CHAPTER 63

Postinflammatory Hypopigmentation (ICD-9 709.00)

Jeffrey P. Callen, M.D.

SYMPTOMS AND SIGNS

Generally, postinflammatory hypopigmentation is asymptomatic unless there is still an existing inflammatory disorder elsewhere. Patients with darker skin are more prone to develop this condition. The inflammatory reaction that precedes the reaction may be intense and obvious, or it may be subtle and barely even noticed by the patient. The problem is a common sequela of eczema (Fig. 63-1). Mild atopic dermatitis can result in pityriasis alba, hypopigmented patches on the face most commonly seen in African-American children. Hypopigmentation frequently follows cutaneous lupus erythematosus, both in chronic and subacute forms, and lichen planus.

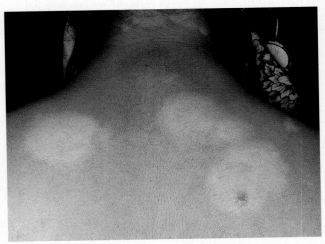

FIGURE 1. Postinflammatory hypopigmentation due to eczema.

DIFFERENTIAL DIAGNOSIS

Vitiligo is due to total loss, not simply a decrease, in pigmentation. Under the Wood's lamp, its border is sharply defined, and there is no pigmentation. Postinflammatory hypopigmentation is ill defined, and there is evidence of incomplete pigment loss.

HOW TO MAKE THE DIAGNOSIS

Postinflammatory hypopigmentation can usually be diagnosed on clinical examination. Punch biopsy is helpful at times in determining the cause of the hypopigmentation.

THERAPY

Therapy for the causative condition of postinflammatory hypopigmentation aids in prevention of additional lesions. In many cases, the pigmentation returns. But generally, darker patients take longer to repigment. Because pityriasis alba has subtle continued inflammation, a low- to medium-potent topical corticosteroid may be helpful.

PROGNOSIS

Postinflammatory hypopigmentation has, by itself, no implied prognosis. The prognosis is directly linked to the disease that caused it.

CHAPTER 64
Lichen Sclerosus et Atrophicus
(ICD-9 701.0)
Jeffrey P. Callen, M.D.

SYMPTOMS AND SIGNS

Patients with lichen sclerosus et atrophicus (LS&A) complain of rough or dry patches of skin that are sometimes pruritic. Genital lesions cause sexual dysfunction and dyspareunia. LS&A presents commonly as kraurosis vulvae, a keyhole or "figure 8" configuration of well-demarcated, hypopigmented, slightly atrophic patches around the vulva and perineum (Fig. 64-1). Skin atrophy is common; the surface is shiny and wrinkles like cigarette paper. Lesions on the penis are called **balanitis xerotica obliterans.**

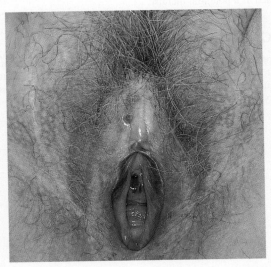

FIGURE 1. Lichen sclerosus et atrophicus. Kraurosis vulvae with "keyhole" configuration around the vulva and perineum.

DIFFERENTIAL DIAGNOSIS

At times, LS&A overlaps with morphea (localized scleroderma) in the same patient. Genital lesions of lichen planus are often violaceous and erosive and are accompanied by lesions on the skin or mucous mem-

159

branes or both. The possibility of sexual abuse is considered when hemorrhage occurs in genital lesions.

HOW TO MAKE THE DIAGNOSIS

Clinical suspicion of LS&A is confirmed by punch biopsy.

THERAPY

Despite the fact that LS&A appears to be an atrophic process, superpotent topical corticosteroid ointments are highly effective. When topical steroids are used on the genitalia, topical anticandidal therapy may also be needed to prevent secondary yeast infection. Topical testosterone has been used in the past, but this therapy is ineffective and often associated with androgenic toxic effects. Therefore, it should be discarded as a potential therapy.

PROGNOSIS

Some patients have spontaneous resolution of LS&A, particularly children. It has been believed that genital lesions may be associated with subsequent development of squamous cell carcinoma, but this is a controversy that has not been resolved.

CHAPTER 65

Vitiligo (ICD-9 709.1)

Jeffrey P. Callen, M.D.

SYMPTOMS AND SIGNS

Vitiligo is usually asymptomatic, but because the depigmented skin is very sensitive to sunlight, patients may complain of sunburn. Periorificial depigmentation is observed early in the course (Fig. 65-1). Acral areas are commonly affected. Depigmented areas are sharply demarcated from adjacent, normally pigmented skin. Vitiligo can begin at any age, but it most commonly begins in adolescence or young adulthood. The disease is believed to be the result of an autoimmune disorder that targets the melanocyte, and it is not uncommon for patients to have associated autoimmune disorders, such as thyroiditis, pernicious anemia, and alopecia areata.

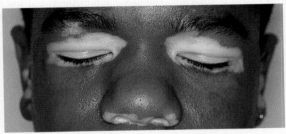

FIGURE 1. Periorificial vitiligo showing sharp demarcations between normally pigmented and depigmented skin.

DIFFERENTIAL DIAGNOSIS

In postinflammatory hypopigmentation, there is usually a history of a preexisting inflammatory skin disorder such as eczema or lichen planus. Wood's light examination demonstrates only partial loss of pigment. Piebaldism is congenital, localized, and nonprogressive and there are multiple color variations. Hydroquinone-containing products and some other chemicals can cause pigment loss.

HOW TO MAKE THE DIAGNOSIS

The diagnosis of vitiligo is clinical. Punch biopsy is rarely needed. After the diagnosis is established, patients should be assessed for associated conditions by thyroid function tests and a complete blood count.

THERAPY

Medium-potent or high-potent topical corticosteroid ointments or creams may be effective. Although vitiliginous skin seems less prone to atrophy from topical steroids, reevaluation should occur every 4 to 6 weeks and include a Wood's light examination. Therapeutic response is usually noted within 2 to 3 months and often begins in a perifollicular pattern. PUVA therapy, UVA light combined with oral or topical psoralen—a photosensitizing agent—is another approach. PUVA therapy is administered two to three times weekly in a controlled setting under the direction of a physician. It often takes 6 to 8 weeks to begin to take effect. Sending patients to tanning facilities is not advisable.

PROGNOSIS

Vitiligo is difficult to treat. Because the skin lacks pigment, it is more prone to sunburn. Therefore, sun protection methods and sun blocks should be used. Patients should be assessed for skin cancer regularly.

CHAPTER 66

Morphea (Localized Scleroderma)

(ICD-9 701.1)

Jeffrey P. Callen, M.D.

SYMPTOMS AND SIGNS

Morphea (localized scleroderma) is an asymptomatic condition limited to the skin. Some patients complain of a tight feeling of their skin, or pruritus or burning. Morphea is a localized hardening of the skin. The condition occurs in three forms—plaques, linear, and generalized. Plaques of morphea are indurated and red to violaceous at their borders (Fig. 66-1). Linear scleroderma (morphea) has a similar appearance. It occurs on the face, where it is known as "en coup de sabre," or on the extremities. Facial linear scleroderma may rarely affect underlying tissues including the bones and the brain. In generalized morphea, plaques are large and widespread.

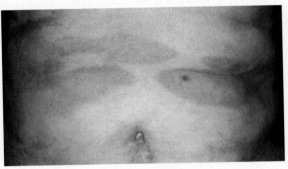

FIGURE 1. Morphea. Extensive hyperpigmented and violaceous plaques.

DIFFERENTIAL DIAGNOSIS

Localized scars usually have a history of trauma. Systemic scleroderma (progressive systemic sclerosis) is characterized by sclerodactyly, Raynaud's phenomenon, and systemic involvement manifested as dysphagia, arthritis, and dyspnea.

HOW TO MAKE THE DIAGNOSIS

The diagnosis of morphea is clinical, but it is useful to have a punch biopsy for confirmation. Laboratory abnormalities are relatively uncommon in localized scleroderma with the exception of a positive antinuclear antibody test (40% to 50%) and frequently the presence of antihistone antibodies (25% to 50%).

THERAPY

There is no uniformly accepted therapy for morphea. In fact, it is not clear that any of the proposed therapies work. Patients with overlapping features of lichen sclerosus et atrophicus may respond to superpotent topical corticosteroid ointments or creams. Topical calcipotriene cream or ointment 0.005% once or twice daily under occlusion has been reported to be effective. Physical therapy helps patients with joint deformities.

PROGNOSIS

Over months to years, most patients have spontaneous softening of affected areas. Those with facial hematrophy may be left with permanent disfigurement, and those with lesions occurring over joints may have contractures.

CHAPTER 67

Scleroderma (Progressive Systemic Sclerosis) (ICD-9 701.0)

Jeffrey P. Callen, M.D.

SYMPTOMS AND SIGNS

The onset of scleroderma [progressive systemic sclerosis (PSS)] is insidious. Patients often complain first of Raynaud's phenomenon. The skin in PSS is taut and bound down. It is shiny and may become dyspigmented. The disease may be limited or diffuse. The limited form of PSS is more common and is characterized by a slowly progressive hardening of the acral skin, known as sclerodactyly (Fig. 67-1). In diffuse PSS, sclerodactyly is accompanied by widespread involvement of both the skin and the internal organs. Systemic symptoms include fatigue, dysphagia, dyspnea, abnormal bowel function, arthralgias, and myalgias. Hypertension may be caused by PSS involving the kidneys. A variant, known as the **CREST syndrome,** is characterized by calcinosis, Raynaud's phenomenon, esophageal dysmotility, sclerodactyly, and telangiectasia.

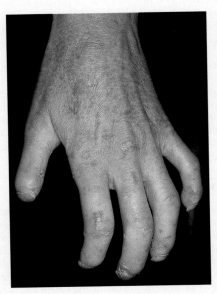

FIGURE 1. Scleroderma. Sclerodactyly; taut, bound-down skin on hands.

DIFFERENTIAL DIAGNOSIS

Morphea (localized scleroderma) is a distinct and separate disease causing localized areas of induration. Eosinophilic fasciitis (EF), which is rare, causes a rapid onset of proximal sclerosis without associated Raynaud's phenomenon. EF patients have eosinophilia and hyperglobulinemia. The clinical manifestations characteristically begin after an episode of excessive exertion. Eosinophilia myalgia syndrome has similar features to those of EF, but is triggered by contaminated L-tryptophan.

HOW TO MAKE THE DIAGNOSIS

Scleroderma is diagnosed by a constellation of findings after the exclusion of other diseases. Once diagnosed, the patient should be assessed for severity of the disease. Laboratory evaluation includes serologic tests for antinuclear antibodies, anticentromere antibody (ACA), and antitopoisomerase I (Scl-70) antibody. The ACA is common in patients with the CREST variant (80% to 90%). Scl-70 indicates diffuse and often rapidly progressive PSS. Patients also should have esophageal motility studies if they complain of dysphagia and they should have upper gastrointestinal x-rays with bowel follow through if they have other gastrointestinal symptoms. Chest x-ray and pulmonary function tests should be performed in all patients because of the high rate of asymptomatic pulmonary dysfunction.

THERAPY

There is no cure for PSS. It is not clear that the process can be arrested or reversed. D-penicillamine and extracorporeal photopheresis are controversial. Nonspecific therapy is directed at the symptoms and signs such as calcium channel blockers (nifedipine 30 to 60 mg daily by mouth) or topical nitroglycerin for Raynaud's phenomenon, nonsteroidal antiinflammatory drugs for arthralgias and myalgias, and elevation of the head during sleep to prevent aspiration for patients with esophageal dysmotility.

PROGNOSIS

The prognosis of patients with PSS is dependent on the presence of systemic disease. Although patients with renal involvement represent less than 5%, about 30% to 50% have rapidly progressive and life-threatening disease. In the absence of renal disease, scleroderma is slowly progressive, and the presence and severity of cardiopulmonary involvement determines the outcome. Survival of patients with the CREST variant can be 10 to 20 years in the absence of progressive pulmonary dysfunction.

CHAPTER 68

Lentigo (ICD-9 709.0)

Charles A. Gropper, M.D.

SYMPTOMS AND SIGNS

Lentigines are asymptomatic small, brown macules. There are three major types: lentigo simplex, solar lentigo, and lentigo maligna.

Lentigo simplex may occur anywhere on the skin or mucous membranes. It is a small macule, about 1 to 8 mm in diameter, tan to dark brown or black, and uniformly pigmented. Lentigo simplex is not related to sun exposure. In Peutz–Jeghers syndrome, simple lentigines are associated with polyps of the gastrointestinal tract and increased risk of gastrointestinal or genitourinary carcinoma (Fig. 68-1).

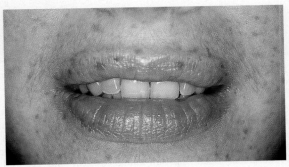

FIGURE 1. Simple lentigo on the lips of a patient with Peutz–Jeghers syndrome.

Solar lentigo, known by the lay term "liver spot," have a similar appearance to that of lentigo simplex, but are induced by sunlight. They develop on sun-exposed areas, usually in older people, and can be larger than lentigo simplex, up to 2 cm in diameter.

Lentigo maligna is a large brown patch with irregular pigment and shape on sun-damaged skin (Fig. 68-2). It is most common in patients over the age of 60. Approximately 5% of lentigo malignas progress to lentigo maligna melanoma; it is therefore sometimes referred to as malignant melanoma in situ.

DIFFERENTIAL DIAGNOSIS

Unlike freckles, lentigines do not darken with sunlight and can occur anywhere on the body, including the mucous membranes.

167

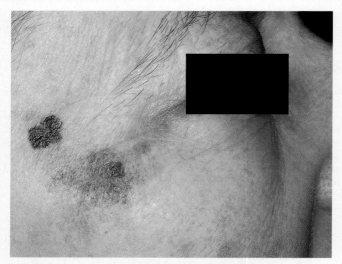

FIGURE 2. Lentigo maligna with irregular borders and variable pigmentation on sun-exposed skin (one lesion).

Junctional nevi can appear identical with lentigines on examination and sometimes can only be differentiated on biopsy. Nevi and flat seborrheic keratoses frequently have a bumpy surface. Pigmented actinic keratoses occur on sun-damaged skin and are red and scaling. Lentigo maligna must be distinguished from lentigo maligna melanoma by punch or excisional biopsy. Lentigo maligna appears on sun-damaged skin and has markedly irregular pigment and irregular borders. Lentigo maligna melanoma has similar findings, but variability of color and border irregularity are more pronounced.

HOW TO MAKE THE DIAGNOSIS

Diagnosis of lentigines is often clinical, but excisional biopsy must be done if malignant melanoma is suspected.

TREATMENT

Lentigo simplex and solar lentigines are treated mainly for cosmetic reasons. Lentigines that are very dark in color should be biopsied to rule out melanocytic atypia. Lentigo simplex and solar lentigo can be treated with cryotherapy, tretinoin cream 0.025% daily, or surgical excision. Sunscreens and sun avoidance can be helpful for solar lentigines.

Surgical excision is the most effective treatment for lentigo maligna, but more conservative treatments such as cryotherapy or electrodesiccation and curettage may be sufficient.

PROGNOSIS

Lentigo simplex and solar lentigines are benign lesions. They usually persist throughout life, though a small number will fade or disappear. In contrast, lentigo maligna is a lesion with known premalignant potential. Malignant degeneration of lentigo maligna usually occurs in lesions that have been present for more than 10 years. Since approximately 5% of lentigo maligna lesions will progress to lentigo maligna melanoma, they must be followed closely with a bias towards early biopsy and treatment.

CHAPTER 69

Postinflammatory Hyperpigmentation (ICD-9 709.00)

Charles A. Gropper, M.D.

SYMPTOMS AND SIGNS

Patients often complain of an asymptomatic dark spot or patch on the skin that seemed to appear "out of nowhere." The spot may have blurred borders and may be irregularly shaped (Fig. 69-1; see Fig. 2-2). Since any inflammatory dermatosis can heal with hyperpigmentation, the diagnosis is suggested by the history of a preceding rash that has evolved into a darker hue in the same distribution. Patients often are concerned that the darkening of color indicates a worsening of their condition; they need reassurance that the color change is actually part of the healing process.

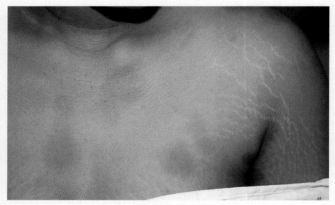

FIGURE 1. Postinflammatory hyperpigmentation due to eczema.

HOW TO MAKE THE DIAGNOSIS

The diagnosis of postinflammatory hyperpigmentation is established by history of prior inflammatory dermatosis and clinical appearance.

DIFFERENTIAL DIAGNOSIS

Melasma appears in a symmetric distribution on the cheeks and is frequently associated with pregnancy. In acanthosis nigricans, the skin surface is usually bumpy and scaly, and the condition is limited to the axillae, posterior neck, and groin. Patients who have used bleaching creams with hydroquinones can develop exogenous ochronosis characterized by intensely dark patches on the affected areas.

TREATMENT

Identification and treatment of the inflammatory dermatosis that caused the hyperpigmentation is an important first step. Treatment is difficult; it is hard to predict which patients will respond and how well they will respond. There are several treatment options. All are most helpful if applied within the first 2 months of the development of hyperpigmentation.

Bleaching creams containing 4% hydroquinone may be effective if the pigment is very superficial and confined to the epidermis. Alternatives include high-potency topical corticosteroid ointments or creams applied daily, or tretinoin cream 0.05% applied each night. Patients should be encouraged to use sun block with SPF of at least 15 to decrease the chances of further hyperpigmentation due to sunlight.

PROGNOSIS

Postinflammatory hyperpigmentation may take months or years to disappear.

CHAPTER 70
Leg Ulcers (ICD-9 707.1)
John T. Crissey, M.D.

SYMPTOMS AND SIGNS

Venous Ulcers (Stasis Ulcers)

Venous ulcers are more common in women; patients are usually middle-aged or older, often with a history of thrombophlebitis. Although pain and tenderness associated with venous ulcers may be pronounced, symptoms are usually less prominent than one might expect from the clinical appearance.

Venous ulcers often follow a minor injury. They are usually unilateral, involving the lower third of the leg and ankle, especially the malleoli. Borders are sharp and often irregular. The surrounding skin may be markedly thickened, hyperpigmented, and pebbly. Chronic lymphedema is also often present. The base of the ulcer, which bleeds easily when disturbed, is made up of granulation tissue and necrotic slough in varying proportions (Fig. 70-1).

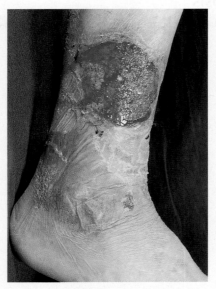

FIGURE 1. Venous stasis ulcer on lower leg with bleeding, granulation tissue with surrounding venous stasis changes.

Signs of chronic venous insufficiency in the areas surrounding the ulcers provide clues to the diagnosis: red-brown speckles of hemosiderosis against the more uniformly brownish background of hyperpigmentation, along with scattered purpuric macules. Eczematous changes—patchy areas of brighter erythema, moist papules, scaling, serous crusting, and excoriations—may also be present.

Arterial Ulcers (Ischemic Ulcers)

Atherosclerosis is the usual cause of arterial ulcer (AU) in the elderly. Men are more susceptible than women. AUs are uncommon before middle life. Pain is the outstanding feature, and intermittent claudication is often prominent. Arterial ulcers are usually sharply defined and round, as if punched out (Fig. 70-2). They tend to be smaller than venous ulcers and may be deep enough to expose muscle and tendons. The base is commonly covered with a necrotic slough. Pretibial areas, toes, and dorsa of the feet are the favored sites.

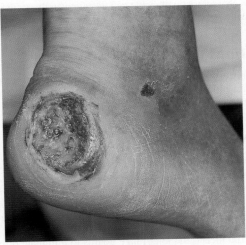

FIGURE 2. Arterial ulcer with sharp borders in a patient with poor circulation due to diabetes.

Changes in the skin of the legs, ankles, and feet provide clues to the diagnosis of AU. There is pallor and often cyanosis, sometimes accompanied by the mottled violaceous erythema known as livedo reticularis. The pallor is especially evident when the leg is elevated.

Changes are usually bilateral. The legs and feet have a cold, clammy feel. Thickening and distortion of the toenails (onychogryphosis) and absence of arterial pulses are common signs as well.

DIFFERENTIAL DIAGNOSIS

When leg ulcers occur in the absence of either venous or arterial insufficiency, the cause is usually a bacterial infection preceded by a traumatic episode. Ulcers belonging to this group can be located anywhere on the leg and are seldom more than 3 or 4 cm in diameter. They are usually tender and are often surrounded by a prominent zone of erythema. Bacterial and fungal cultures are indicated when vascular problems are absent. Punch biopsy of the border of the lesion is helpful in these cases. Special stains can be used to identify fungi and other microorganisms or to identify neoplastic disease, which is also an occasional cause. Streptococci, staphylococci (especially enterococci), mycobacteria, *Treponema pallidum,* and *Leishmani donovani* all are capable of producing ulcers on the legs. The punched-out ulcers about the ankles characteristic of sickle cell disease usually occur in younger patients, who show no signs of venous or arterial insufficiency.

HOW TO MAKE A DIAGNOSIS

Note the history and morphology, check for circulatory problems, and culture and biopsy the ulcer border if circulation appears normal. Biopsy material should be stained for bacteria and fungi.

TREATMENT

Treatments of venous ulcers are largely strategies for improving venous return: leg elevation, elastic stockings and roll bandages, and surgical intervention (ligation and stripping procedures). Grafting is sometimes feasible. Eczematous eruptions (stasis dermatitis) usually improve with medium-, high- or super-potent topical corticosteroid ointments or creams.

For arterial ulcers, the long-range goal is to eliminate or control as many of the major risk factors associated with peripheral vascular disease as possible, namely smoking, hypertension, hyperlipoproteinemia, obesity, and diabetes mellitus. Foot care is of great importance. Corns, callosities, and nail dystrophies merit professional attention. Pharmacologic treatment, although often disappointing, is worth trying. Pentoxifylline has produced beneficial results in some cases at a dosage of 400 mg three times daily by mouth (with meals). Surgical consultation is indicated in every case. Distal arterial bypass grafting or lumbar sympathectomy may offer the best or only chance to pre-serve a severely compromised extremity.

Treatment of leg ulcers that are not circulatory in origin must be tai-lored to the cause.

PROGNOSIS

Venous ulcers tend to be chronic. Compliance with therapy and pre-ventive measures can significantly improve prognosis. Prognosis in ar-terial ulcers is guarded. Surgical intervention offers the best hope for successful outcome.

CHAPTER 71

Onychomycosis (ICD-9 110.9)

Charles A. Gropper, M.D.

SYMPTOMS AND SIGNS

Onychomycosis is usually asymptomatic. Sometimes, however, it is painful, especially when there is secondary bacterial infection or when the dystrophic growth pattern causes an ingrown toenail. In a small number of extremely severe cases, there can be difficulty in ambulation. Affected nails become yellow, thickened, and onycholytic, meaning that the nail plate partially separates from the nail bed (Fig. 71-1). Toenails are more often affected than fingernails; one common pattern is both feet infected, but only one hand. It is common for only some nails on a foot or hand to be involved, whereas neighboring nails are spared.

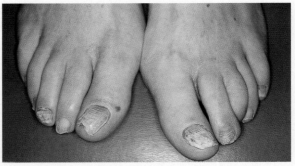

FIGURE 1. Yellow, thickened, and onycholytic toenails due to *Trichophyton rubrum*.

Onychomycosis is extremely common. Total prevalence in the United States is in the range of 5% to 10%, and up to 20% of people over age 40 will have this problem at some point in their lives. The most common agent is *Trichophyton rubrum*.

DIFFERENTIAL DIAGNOSIS

Psoriatic nails can appear identical with nails with onychomycosis, with yellowing, hyperkeratosis, and onychocholysis. Psoriatic nails may have additional clinical features such as pitting and "oil spots," which are yellow-brown spots under the nail plate. The presence of

176

typical psoriatic plaques on other parts of the body suggests the diagnosis of psoriasis.

HOW TO MAKE THE DIAGNOSIS

The clinical diagnosis of onychomycosis can be confirmed by identifying fungal elements in a 10% potassium hydroxide preparation of nail plate scales. Alternatively, nail clippings may be sent to the laboratory for fungal culture, but results take weeks to arrive. Neither of these tests is positive in 100% of cases, so clinical impression must be the final arbiter of diagnosis.

TREATMENT

Until recently, the mainstay of treatment for onychomycosis was at least 1 year of therapy with griseofulvin. Even then, the success rate was only about 30%, and the relapse rate was over 50%. Topical antifungal preparations are ineffective in the treatment of onychomycosis. The availability of two new oral agents, terbinafine and itraconazole, has greatly improved treatment options. Terbinafine, 250 mg daily, is given for 6 weeks for fingernails and 12 weeks for toenails. Itraconazole can be given as a "pulse dose," in which the patient takes 200 mg twice daily for 1 week of each month. This regimen is followed 2 months for fingernails and 3 months for toenails.

Liver function tests should be checked before either treatment and rechecked 1 month after treatment begins.

PROGNOSIS

With terbinafine and itraconazole, onychomycosis is cured in about 80% of patients. Patients must be reminded that nail growth is slow. The full effect of treatment is not seen until 6 to 8 months in fingernails and 9 to 12 months for toenails. Relapse rate is about 15% within 18 months of treatment.

CHAPTER 72

Pseudomonas Nails (ICD-9 041.7)

Charles A. Gropper, M.D.

SYMPTOMS AND SIGNS

Patients with *Pseudomonas aeruginosa* infection of the nail plate complain of blue-green changes or of a sickly sweet, "fruity" smell similar to that of rotting grapes (Fig. 72-1). The blue-green pattern may occur in sequential transverse bands reflecting intermittent intensity of infection. Sometimes, the paronychial areas swell. In general, this is an indolent condition. This problem occurs in people whose hands are frequently wet.

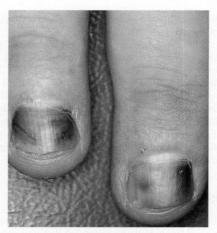

FIGURE 1. Green nails due to *Pseudomonas aeruginosa* infection.

DIFFERENTIAL DIAGNOSIS

Dermatophyte infections turn nails yellow.

HOW TO MAKE THE DIAGNOSIS

The diagnosis of *Pseudomonas* nails is made on the characteristic appearance and odor. Culture of involved nail plates sometimes confirms the diagnosis.

TREATMENT

Nails usually respond rapidly to topical or systemic antibiotics that offer good gram-negative coverage. A good choice is ciprofloxacin, 750 mg twice daily by mouth for 10 days.

PROGNOSIS

Fingernails will appear normal 3 to 6 months after the active infection has been eradicated. For toenails, the wait may be twice as long.

CHAPTER 73

Acute (ICD-9 112.3) and Chronic Paronychia (ICD-9 681.02)

Charles A. Gropper, M.D.

SYMPTOMS AND SIGNS

Acute paronychia is a very painful and tender infection of the proximal and lateral nail folds. It is usually caused by *Staphylococcus aureus*; occasionally, group A streptococci, and gram-negative bacteria are responsible. The nail folds become red and swollen, and there may be frank drainage of pus (Fig. 73-1). After several months, the nail may break (onycholysis) or become ridged. Acute paronychia occurs frequently in diabetics and in patients who are immunocompromised.

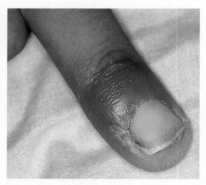

FIGURE 1. Acute paronychia with tender, red, swollen proximal and lateral nail folds.

Chronic paronychia has a less dramatic presentation and is often due to *Candida albicans.* Contact dermatitis, fixed drug eruptions, psoriasis, and dyshidrotic eczema also cause chronic paronychia. Repeated hand trauma or washing leads to a loss of the seal between the nail plate and nail folds, and infectious or irritative agents can gain entry. Dentists, bakers, and construction workers are often affected.

DIFFERENTIAL DIAGNOSIS

Nail-fold welling and erythema of herpetic whitlow often extends to the finger, and Tzanck smear or viral culture confirms the diagnosis. Neoplasms of the nail matrix are usually painless. Careful examination shows a narrow band of alteration of the nail plate, reflecting the focal location of the lesion within the nail matrix. A history of psoriasis or eczema, along with characteristic lesions on other parts of the body suggests these diagnoses.

HOW TO MAKE THE DIAGNOSIS

The significant pain and the clinical appearance of paronychia make the diagnosis. Culture may demonstrate responsible organisms.

TREATMENT

Severe, painful acute paronychia may require lancing with a No. 11 blade to release the purulent fluid accumulating under the nail fold. Patients who require lancing should always be treated with antistaphylococcal antibiotics for at least 7 days. In chronic paronychia due to *Candida*, lancing is not indicated. Topical therapy, such as imidazole cream (see Chapter 23) or 2% to 4% thymol in chloroform (or absolute alcohol) two to three times daily may suffice. In severe cases, an oral agent such as itraconazole, 200 mg daily for 7 days, may be necessary. Because chronic paronychia is often superinfected with bacteria, a course of antistaphylococcal antibiotics may also be necessary.

PROGNOSIS

Infection tends to be recurrent, especially in patients who are unable to avoid frequent hand washing. Patients can be advised to wear light cotton gloves under their work gloves. They also should avoid direct contact with irritants, where possible. Resolution of nail changes may take up to 6 months after an infection is resolved.

CHAPTER 74

Alopecia Areata (ICD-9 704.01)

Charles A. Gropper, M.D.

SYMPTOMS AND SIGNS

In alopecia areata (AA), round patches of hair loss develop rapidly and asymptomatically. The patches are well-circumscribed, round, and without inflammation or scarring (Fig. 74-1). Hair loss occurs most commonly on the scalp, but other areas such as the eyebrows and beard are often involved. AA is a chronic, recurrent condition that often begins in childhood or in young adults. The term **alopecia totalis** is used

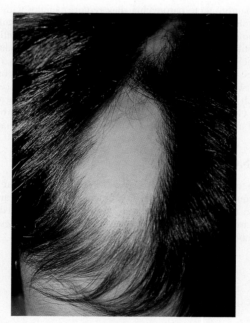

FIGURE 1. Alopecia areata. Patches of alopecia are well circumscribed, round, and without inflammation.

if all scalp hair is lost, and **alopecia universalis** is the term for complete loss of all body hair. As much as 1% of the population may have at least one spot of AA by age 50. There is a positive family history of AA in 10% to 20% of patients.

One pathognomonic sign of AA is the "exclamation point" hair, which is wide distally and narrow at the base and occurs at the periphery of a patch of hair loss (Fig. 74-2). Hairs that regrow in a patch of AA often are white. Pitting of the nails accompanies hair loss in about 40% of patients. Most patients are in good health, and no additional medical workup is required. In a small number of cases, however, there is an association with other autoimmune conditions such as Hashimoto's thyroiditis, connective tissue disease, myasthenia gravis, cataracts, and vitiligo.

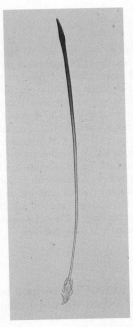

FIGURE 2. Alopecia areata. Exclamation point hairs are wide distally and narrow at the base.

DIFFERENTIAL DIAGNOSIS

In tinea capitis, there is scaling and erythema. Trichotillomania appears in an irregular-shaped patch of hair loss, not well circumscribed as in AA, with some of the hairs having broken ends. The patient may also have a history of hair trauma and petechiae on the scalp around follicles. Androgenetic alopecia involves most of the scalp rather than small round patches and occurs in characteristic male or female patterns.

HOW TO MAKE THE DIAGNOSIS

The presence of well-demarcated, round patches of nonscarring alopecia is characteristic. Exclamation point hairs and nail pitting, when present, are helpful in confirming the diagnosis of AA (see Fig. 74-2). Punch biopsy is usually not needed to rule out other causes.

TREATMENT

AA has a variable course, and new lesions may develop even as old ones are resolving. This makes evaluation of treatments difficult, and no treatment has been extremely effective. The main treatment option in AA is intralesional injection of dilute glucocorticosteroids such as triamcinolone acetonide suspension in a concentration of 2.5 to 5 mg/mL. Injections are given every 3 to 4 weeks. Total dose per treatment session should not exceed 20 mg. Topical corticosteroid ointments or creams may be used as an additional treatment, but efficacy is marginal. It is best to use high-potent topical corticosteroids, although results are marginal. These steroids can be used for weeks to months, but skin atrophy is a concern with prolonged use. Topical anthralin, which elicits a mild contact immune response, has been used with modest success. The cream is applied nightly, in a concentration starting at 0.1% and increasing to 1% as tolerated. Minoxidil solution 2% or 5% is of mild benefit in some patients.

PROGNOSIS

About 33% of patients with AA have complete hair regrowth within 1 year. Eighty percent of patients who first develop this condition after puberty eventually have complete regrowth. Complete regrowth is even more assured in children. Poor prognostic signs include involvement of the occipital region, repeated attacks, nail changes, and total alopecia before puberty.

CHAPTER 75

Androgenetic Alopecia (ICD-9 704.00)

Charles A. Gropper, M.D.

SYMPTOMS AND SIGNS

Androgenetic alopecia is asymptomatic but often causes great psychological distress. Hair loss is gradual, and there are no surface changes on the scalp. The hairs become shorter and narrower and eventually fall out. In men, the frontotemporal scalp and vertex are most commonly involved, and progression to complete hair loss may occur. In general, hair density must decline about 15% before it is noticed.

Women also experience androgenetic alopecia. Unlike in men, however, the pattern is more diffuse, although hair loss on the crown is common (Fig. 75-1). Women only rarely develop male-pattern frontotemporal alopecia, and complete hair loss is rare.

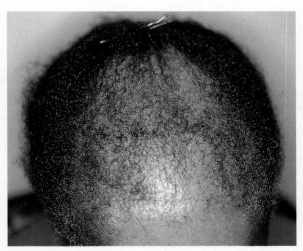

FIGURE 1. Diffuse hair loss in a woman with androgenetic alopecia

DIFFERENTIAL DIAGNOSIS

It is helpful in any case of hair loss to distinguish between scarring and nonscarring diseases. Examine the follicles carefully. Scarring alopecia is characterized by disruption of follicles, in some cases with crust, erosion, or thickening of the scalp. The presence of scarring alopecia suggests diagnoses such as lupus erythematosus or dissecting cellulitis. Nonscarring alopecia points toward medical causes of hair loss, such as androgenetic alopecia, telogen effluvium, alopecia areata, and thyroid dysfunction. Medications causing alopecia include oral contraceptives, coumarin, heparin, propranolol, and vitamin A.

Telogen effluvium tends to involve the entire scalp uniformly and follows a period of stress by 3 to 6 months. Alopecia areata presents with well-circumscribed, round patches of hair loss. Secondary syphilis appears as a patchy, "moth-eaten" alopecia and should be associated with other findings, such as scaly rash, mucous patches, and condyloma latum.

HOW TO MAKE THE DIAGNOSIS

The diagnosis of androgenetic alopecia is made by the history of gradual, progressive loss of hair in the characteristic distribution. Punch biopsy is usually not necessary to confirm the diagnosis.

TREATMENT

For men, two treatments are now available, which have limited benefit. Minoxidil solution, 2% or 5% applied twice daily, results in decrease of hair shedding in about 80% of patients. Up to 60% of patients experience at least minimal regrowth of hair within 12 months of commencing treatment. With finasteride, 1 mg daily by mouth, 80% of men will have the same or a greater amount of hair after 2 years of therapy, and 65% will have at least some visible regrowth. The drug may cause decreased libido, erectile dysfunction, and ejaculation disorders in about 2% of patients.

For women, minoxidil solution 2% applied twice daily brings results similar to those seen in men. Finasteride is contraindicated in women; it is dangerous for pregnant women to touch the pills because of a risk of genital malformations in the fetus.

PROGNOSIS

Progression of androgenetic alopecia is unpredictable.

CHAPTER 76

Telogen Effluvium (ICD-9 704.02)

Charles A. Gropper, M.D.

SYMPTOMS AND SIGNS

Telogen effluvium is asymptomatic. Hair loss in telogen effluvium is evenly distributed throughout the scalp. About 30% to 50% of the scalp hair is involved, so patients do retain a fairly full head of hair even during the worst of the shedding process (Fig. 76-1). There is no scarring. Sometimes referred to as telogen defluvium, the condition is a sudden diffuse loss of scalp hair occurring 3 to 6 months after a stressful event, such as systemic illness or pregnancy. The hair loss is caused by the simultaneous cycling of an unusually high percentage of scalp hairs into the resting, or telogen, phase. Normally, about 5% to 10% of hairs are in the telogen phase; during telogen effluvium, this number increases to about 30%. Normally, resting hairs are retained in the scalp for about 80 to 100 days until they are shed. This explains the 3- to 6-month delay in the development of clinically apparent hair loss after the stressful event. Additional causes of telogen effluvium include neoplasms, infections, and crash diets. Some medications have also been implicated, including heparin, coumarin, propanolol, haloperidol, and lithium.

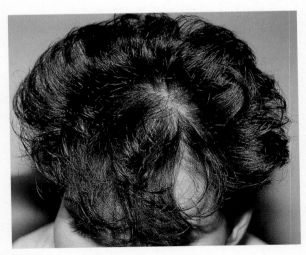

FIGURE 1. Telogen effluvium after pregnancy.

187

DIFFERENTIAL DIAGNOSIS

In androgenetic alopecia or alopecia areata, the areas of hair are well circumscribed and not diffuse in contrast to telogen effluvium.

HOW TO MAKE THE DIAGNOSIS

The diagnosis of telogen effluvium is suggested by the history of a recent stressful event. A hair pull test reveals greater than normal numbers of telogen hairs with clubbed ends. In patients with telogen effluvium, about 50% of hairs have the clubbed ends; in normal patients, only 10% of hairs are clubbed.

TREATMENT

No treatment is needed for telogen effluvium aside from reassurance.

PROGNOSIS

In most cases, there is complete regrowth of hair within a few months.

C H A P T E R   7 7

Punch Biopsy

David J. Leffell, M.D.

Equipment needed
❑ Antiseptic solution
❑ 1% lidocaine with/without 1:100,000 epinephrine
    solution
❑ 20% aluminum chloride hexahydrate solution
❑ Biopsy punch (1 to 10 mm diameter)
❑ Iris scissors
❑ Nonabsorbable suture
❑ Needle driver
❑ Syringe and needle
❑ Sterile bandage
❑ Antibiotic ointment
❑ Tissue pathology bottle with formalin

CONSIDERATIONS

Punch biopsy is most helpful in diagnosing skin conditions whose characteristic pathology lies in the dermis. It is the best biopsy technique for undiagnosed rashes and suspected neoplasms.

PROCEDURE

- Prepare the lesion and surrounding skin with antiseptic solution.
- Anesthetize the site with lidocaine 1% with or without epinephrine (1:100,000). Do not use epinephrine on the digits or tip of the penis. It is safe, however, on the nasal tip and ears. Epinephrine can reduce bleeding and make visualization of the lesion easier. The anesthetic effect may be almost immediate, but it is best to wait 3 to 5 minutes before proceeding with the biopsy. The full hemostatic effect takes somewhat longer to occur and helps to maintain hemostasis after the procedure.
- Select the proper punch size. The size depends on the size of the lesion, how much of the lesion (or dermatitis) must be removed to make the histologic diagnosis, its anatomic location, and the differential diagnosis. Punches of 3- and 4-mm diameter are used most often. Disposable punches are more reliably sharp than reusable instruments.
- Gently pinch the skin around the lesion at various angles to determine the direction that the skin stretches and compresses most easily (Fig. 77-1A).

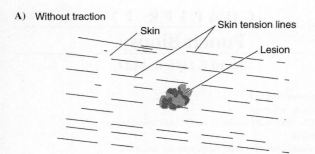

A) Without traction

Skin

Skin tension lines

Lesion

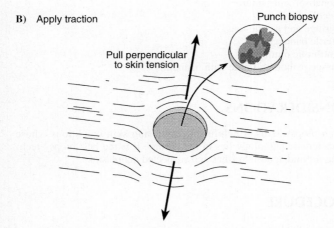

B) Apply traction

Punch biopsy

Pull perpendicular
to skin tension

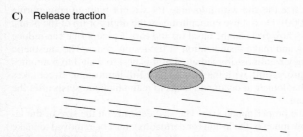

C) Release traction

FIGURE 1. Punch technique, oval wound. **A:** Determine direction that the skin around the lesion stretches and compresses most easily. **B:** Apply tension in direction opposite skin tension lines (*arrows* in direction of tension). **C:** Punch biopsy defect becomes easily sutured oval shape after relaxation of tension.

- Traction should be placed along the axis that most easily was pinched (i.e., perpendicular to the relaxed skin tension lines; see Fig. 77-1B).
- Place the punch atop the lesion and perpendicular to the skin.
- Advance the punch firmly with a gentle pushing and twisting motion that can be clockwise or counterclockwise. As the punch descends through the dermis and into the fat, a "give" is felt as tissue resistance decreases. It is very important not to remove the punch periodically to check the progress or depth. This traumatizes the tissue and may cause histologic artifact.
- Remove the punch only after it enters the fat. Release traction and observe how the circular defect becomes oval and more amenable to suturing (see Fig. 77-1C).
- Lift the tissue sample using a single-prong skin hook or a needle (such as the one used for local anesthesia). The sample must not be crushed or artifact will result.
- Cut the base of the column of tissue with a fine-curved iris scissors, and place the sample in formalin solution in the sample bottle for transport to the pathology laboratory. Be sure to give your dermatopathologist the patient's pertinent history, a description of the lesion, and the differential diagnosis.
- Apply pressure, hemostatic gauze, aluminum chloride solution (or place sutures) to control bleeding. Small defects can heal by second intention, but most wounds heal more rapidly and with a better cosmetic result if closed with simple interrupted or vertical mattress sutures.
- Close the wound. Typically two sutures close a 3- to 4-mm punch biopsy defect.
- Cover the wound with an antibiotic ointment such as polymyxin/bacitracin and a simple sterile dressing.
- Remove sutures on the face in 4 to 7 days. Remove sutures on the trunk in 5 to 7 days; sutures on the extremities should be removed in 7 days.

WOUND CARE INSTRUCTIONS TO PATIENTS

After 24 hours, patients should clean the wound gently daily with soap and tap water. Showering is fine as long as the wound is protected and kept dry.

CHAPTER 78

Shave Biopsy and Shave Excision

David J. Leffell, M.D.

Equipment needed
❏ Antiseptic solution
❏ 1% lidocaine with/without epinephrine 1:100,000 solution
❏ 20% aluminum chloride hexahydrate solution
❏ Sterilized carbon steel razor blade (cut in half lengthwise)
❏ Cotton-tipped applicator
❏ Sterile bandage
❏ Bacitracin/polymyxin ointment

CONSIDERATIONS

Shave biopsy is most helpful for diagnosing diseases where the pathology is in or near the epidermis. Lumps and bumps, as opposed to rashes, are best biopsied with the shave technique. Such lesions appear pedunculated, papular, or exophytic. These include seborrheic keratoses, warts, intradermal nevi, pyogenic granulomas, actinic keratoses, basal cell carcinomas, and squamous cell carcinomas. Lesions suspected of being melanoma should not be biopsied in this manner.

PROCEDURE

- Prepare the lesion and surrounding skin with antiseptic solution.
- Mark the lesion with a sterile marking pen (anesthesia may blur the outlines).
- Anesthetize the site with lidocaine 1% with or without epinephrine (1:100,000). Do not use epinephrine on the digits or on the tip of the penis. It is safe, however, on the nasal tip and ears. Epinephrine can reduce bleeding and make visualization of the lesion easier. The anesthetic effect may be almost immediate but it is best to wait 3 to 5 minutes before proceeding. The full hemostatic effect takes somewhat longer to occur and helps maintain hemostasis after the procedure.
- Hold the flexible, half-razor blade between the thumb and middle or index finger, and remove the lesion with a gentle, forward sawing motion. The depth of excision is determined by the arc of the blade. Note that the blade arc is controlled by pressure placed on the ends of the blade (Fig. 78-1).

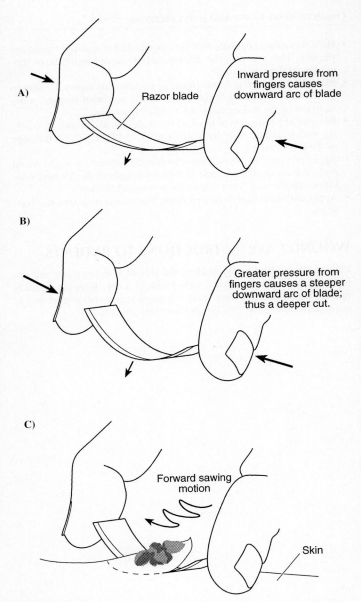

FIGURE 1. A–C: Depth of shave is adjusted by arc of half-razor blade.

193

- Hold down the specimen with the wooden end of a cotton-tipped applicator. This prevents the incompletely removed lesion from flipping away from the blade.
- Place the specimen in formalin and send to the laboratory. Be sure to give the dermatopathologist the patient's pertinent history, a description of the lesion, and a differential diagnosis.
- Remove any remnants of tissue at the margin of the biopsy by scraping with a curette, with the belly of a No. 15 blade, or with the edge of the razor blade.
- Apply pressure, or 20% aluminum chloride solution, or both. Avoid iron-containing styptics such as 20% ferric subsulfate (Monsel's solution) on the face. They can cause permanent tattoos.
- Apply antibiotic ointment, and dress the wound with a sterile bandage.

WOUND CARE INSTRUCTIONS TO PATIENTS

Patients should be advised to clean the wound with tap water and apply antibiotic ointment and a new bandage daily. Keeping wounds open to the air and allowing crust formation retards healing. A moist, occluded wound heals quicker and with less pain.

CHAPTER 79

Cryosurgery

David J. Leffell, M.D.

Equipment needed
- ❏ Liquid nitrogen
- ❏ Liquid nitrogen reservoir (20- to 30-L flask)
- ❏ Paper or polystyrene cup
- ❏ Pressurized spray canister
- ❏ Spray tips and probes of various sizes for canister
- ❏ Cotton-tipped applicators, various sizes
- ❏ Otoscope speculums or neoprene cones

CONSIDERATIONS

Cryosurgery is the therapeutic application of cold, a "controlled frost-bite." Many different cryogens have been used. Liquid nitrogen, at a temperature of $-195.8°$ C ($-320.4°$ F), is the most common. Cryosurgery effectively treats many superficial lesions, such as actinic keratoses, lentigines, molluscum contagiosum, seborrheic keratoses, and warts. Deeper, malignant lesions such as basal cell carcinoma are also treated with cryotherapy, but this requires special equipment and expertise and is not as successful as other methods.

Cryosurgery causes intracellular and extracellular ice crystal formation, alterations in tissue, and vascular stasis. These changes lead to tissue anoxia and necrosis. Melanocytes are most easily destroyed by cryosurgery. This means that hypopigmentation can be a permanent complication of therapy, especially in dark-skinned patients. However, lentigines, for example, can be eliminated without harming the keratinocytes or dermis. Moreover, because fibroblasts are relatively insensitive to cold, scarring rarely follows treatment of superficial lesions.

Cryosurgery can be performed by applying liquid nitrogen with cotton-tipped swabs or by spraying it with the use of a pressurized canister (Fig. 79-1). For either technique, a fast freeze and a slow thaw cause the greatest amount of tissue damage. The extent of tissue damage depends on the pressure, duration of application, and the number of freeze-thaw cycles.

PROCEDURE

Application Technique

- Tease and twist the end of a cotton-tipped swab so that it is no more than 1 to 2 mm larger than the lesion being treated.

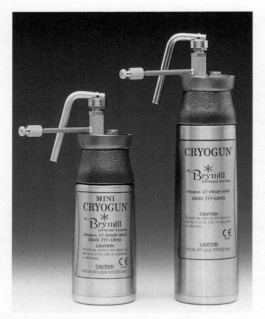

FIGURE 1. Pressurized liquid nitrogen spray canister.

- Dip the swab into the cup of liquid nitrogen, and then hold it firmly against the lesion.
- For thin lesions (such as actinic keratoses and lentigines), 5 to 10 seconds of firm contact should cause formation of an ice ball 1 to 2 mm beyond the margins of the lesion.
- For thicker lesions such as warts and hypertrophic actinic keratoses, the application time is 10 to 30 seconds.

Spray Technique

- Spray the lesion until a full ice ball can be seen. The spray can be controlled with different-sized nozzles supplied with the equipment. Tissue damage can be further controlled by spraying through otoscope speculums or neoprene cones placed around the lesion on the skin. This allows vigorous treatment and deeper damage to the lesion while limiting lateral destruction to surrounding skin.

- For thin lesions, 3 to 5 seconds of continuous spray is adequate.
- For thicker lesions, freeze for 5 to 20 seconds. For deep warts as much as a 60- to 90-second freeze time may be required. A 1- to 3-mm halo of freeze around lesions usually ensures an adequate depth of injury.
- A word of advice: Using many short bursts instead of a few prolonged sprays achieves only minimal tissue penetration. This is inadequate for treating thick lesions. However, it is wise for beginners to err on the side of undertreatment. A partially removed lesion can be retreated, but a scar cannot be eliminated.

WOUND CARE INSTRUCTIONS TO PATIENTS

It is most important to tell patients to expect that superficial lesions will be inflamed for 3 to 7 days and that thicker lesions often blister and contain clear or bloody fluid after treatment. Patients may be taught to sterilize a needle and drain the blister. The roof of the blister should be kept on to serve as an excellent biologic dressing while second-intention healing is underway. Thick lesions take about 2 weeks to heal.

CHAPTER 80

Electrodesiccation and Curettage

David Leffell, M.D.

Equipment needed
- ❏ Antiseptic solution
- ❏ 1% lidocaine with/without epinephrine 1:100,000
  solution
- ❏ Curette (sizes 3 mm to 5 mm)
- ❏ Electrosurgical unit
- ❏ Sterile bandage
- ❏ Bacitracin/polymyxin ointment

CONSIDERATIONS

Electrodesiccation and curettage (EDC) is a useful technique for treating benign, superficial lesions, such as seborrheic keratoses or molluscum contagiosum. EDC can also be used to treat small and superficial basal cell or squamous cell carcinomas. Electrodesiccation refers to directing electric current to the skin surface with a monopolar electrode resulting in destruction of the area. Cell death and tissue necrosis extend beyond the clinically detectable tumor margins, a process that effectively destroys residual malignant cells. EDC is not as effective as excisional surgery for curing basal cell or squamous cell carcinomas. However, the ease of the procedure together with the lower cost and less invasive nature may justify its use when treating small superficial tumors with clearly visible margins.

PROCEDURE

- Prepare the lesion and surrounding skin with antiseptic solution.
- Anesthetize the site with lidocaine 1% with or without epinephrine (1:100,000). Do not use epinephrine on the digits or tip of the penis. It is safe, however, on the nasal tip and ears. Epinephrine can reduce bleeding and make visualization of the lesion easier. The anesthetic effect may be almost immediate, but it is best to wait 3 to 5 minutes before proceeding. The full hemostatic effect takes somewhat longer to occur and helps to maintain hemostasis after the procedure.
- Make sure to anesthetize beyond the visible margins of the lesion because successive cycles of EDC will produce a wider area of tissue damage and charring.
- Start the EDC cycles by initially electrofulgurating the surface. That is, hold the electrode a fraction of a millimeter off the surface of the skin. This effectively removes the epidermal component, which can

then be wiped clean with a gauze pad. Residual cancer is often detectable.

- Curette the tumor gently and extend curettage beyond the obvious area about 3 to 5 mm. Note the difference in feel of the tumor compared with the noninvolved surrounding skin. Basal cell carcinomas tend to feel soft or gelatinous. One can often distinguish the margins of the tumor by feel alone.
- Electrodesiccate the entire base of the curetted area.
- Curette the surface again gently to remove the char, and repeat this cycle up to three times depending on the depth of the tumor.
- The wound bed should be curetted clean with no visible char, active bleeding, or oozing.
- Dress the area with topical antibiotic ointment, and cover the wound with a nonadherent dressing.

WOUND CARE INSTRUCTIONS TO PATIENT

Clean the wound daily with soap and tap water. Apply topical antibiotic ointment and cover the wound under a nonadherent dressing. This should be done until the wound is healed completely. Depending on location, depth of treatment and quality of wound care, this can be from 5 days (locations above the neck) to 14 days (extremities). The healed EDC site may produce a round, hypopigmented, and slightly depressed scar. The scar becomes smaller in time but can be a concern to patients when it is prominent.

Photo Acknowledgments

The following colleagues contributed greatly to the photography in this book. Their photos are used by their permission and as a courtesy; they retain all copyright privileges to their photographs published in this book.

I add a special note of thanks to Drs. Robert J. Cohen (New York University) and Mark G. Lebwohl (Mount Sinai School of Medicine), who generously allowed me to review their vast and excellent collections.

Figures 5-2, 9-1, 32-1 courtesy of Hilary Baldwin.

Figures 4-1, 8-1, 10-1, 13-1, 13-2, 14-1, 14-2, 15-2, 26-1, 30-1, 30-2, 31-1, 31-2, 31-3, 38-1, 60-1, 61-1, 62-1, 63-1, 64-1, 65-1, 66-1, 67-1 courtesy of Jeffrey P. Callen.

Figures 4-2, 20-2, 21-1, 21-2, 23-2, 29-1, 34-1, 35-1, 36-3, 36-4, 37-1, 39-1, 41-1, 42-1, 43-1, 49-1, 50-1, 58-1, 69-1, 74-1, 74-2, 76-1 courtesy of Robert J. Cohen.

Figures 25-1, 25-2, 33-1, 51-1, 54-1, 55-1, 56-1, 59-1, 59-2, 59-3, 70-1 courtesy of John T. Crissey.

Figure 22-2, courtesy of Drore Eisen.

Figure 2-4, courtesy of Annie Fine.

Figures 3-1, 16-1 courtesy of David H. Frankel.

Figures 23-1, 23-3, 24-2 courtesy of Donald Greer.

Figures 40-1, 45-1, 47-1 courtesy of Hossein Nousari.

Figures 9-2, 18-2 courtesy of The Lancet.

Figures 1-1, 6-1, 11-1, 12-1, 20-1, 27-1, 27-2, 44-1, 46-1, 48-1, 52-1, 57-1, 68-1, 70-2, 71-1, 72-1, 73-1, 75-1, courtesy of Mark G. Lebwohl.

Figures 16-2, 17-1, 22-1, 24-1 courtesy of Larry E. Millikan.

Figure 18-1 courtesy of Robert Nadelman.

Figure 15-1 courtesy of Nicholas Soter.

Figures 2-1, 2-2, 2-3, courtesy of Amy Paller.

Figures 4-3, 5-1, 19-1 courtesy of Lawrence Charles Parish.

Figures 8-2, 20-3, 28-3, 36-1, 36-2, 37-2, 39-2, 39-3, 68-2 courtesy of James C. Shaw.

Figures 7-1, 28-1, 28-2, 40-2, 53-1 courtesy of Leonard Swinyer.

Figure 79-1 courtesy of Brymill Cryogenic Systems.

David H. Frankel, M.D.

Subject Index

203

H

Hair
clubbed ends in telogen effluvium, 188
pediculosis capitis and, 16–18

Hair follicle
acne vulgaris and, 26
folliculitis and, 124–125
furuncle and, 131
keratosis pilaris and, 9

Hair loss
in alopecia areata, 64, 182–184
in androgenetic alopecia, 185–186
in dermatomyositis, 39
in secondary syphilis, 70
in telogen effluvium, 187

Hair pull test in telogen effluvium, 188

Halo nevus, 103–104, 109

Halobetasol propionate, 5

Hand
actinic keratosis, 92
atopic dermatitis, 7
dermatomyositis, 39
dyshidrotic eczema, 19
erythema multiforme, 45, 46
granuloma annulare, 122
herpetic whitlow, 76
keratoacanthoma, 94
paronychia, 180–181
Pseudomonas aeruginosa infection of nails, 178–179
psoriatic arthritis, 57
pyogenic granuloma, 126
scabies, 13
sclerodactyly, 165
squamous cell carcinoma, 90
verruca plana, 148
wart, 147
xanthoma, 145

Hand dermatitis, term, 11

Head
actinic keratosis, 92
basal cell carcinoma, 96
discoid lupus erythematosus, 36
seborrheic keratosis, 88

Head louse, 16–18

Heliotrope rash, 39

Herald patch, 59

Herpes simplex virus, 76–78
herpes zoster *versus,* 79

impetigo *versus,* 74
pemphigus vulgaris *versus,* 83

Herpes zoster, 79–81
herpes simplex virus infection *versus,* 77
impetigo *versus,* 74

Herpetic whitlow, 76
paronychia *versus,* 180

Hidradenitis suppurativa, 135–136
furuncle *versus,* 132
squamous cell carcinoma and, 90

Hidrocystoma, 98

High-potent topical corticosteroids, 3, 5

Histamine blockers for urticaria, 44

History
in alopecia areata, 182
in androgenetic alopecia, 186
in chondrodermatitis nodularis chronica helicis, 138
in dermatitis
atopic, 10
contact, 12
in ecchymosis, 153
in erythema multiforme, 47
in generalized pruritus, 25
in halo nevus, 104
in keratoacanthoma, 95
in leg ulcer, 174
in Lyme disease, 51
in postinflammatory hyperpigmentation, 170
in rosacea, 33
in telogen effluvium, 188

Hot tub dermatitis, 124

Human papillomavirus, 147–150

Hydrocortisone
for high-risk areas, 2
over-the-counter preparations, 3
strength and brand name, 5, 6

Hydroxychloroquine
for cutaneous lupus erythematosus, 38
for dermatomyositis, 40–41

Hydroxyzine
for drug eruption, 49
for generalized pruritus, 25
for urticaria, 44

Hyperlinear palm, 7, 8, 10

Hyperpigmentation
in dermatofibroma, 112

Field Guide to
Clinical Dermatology